W0227887

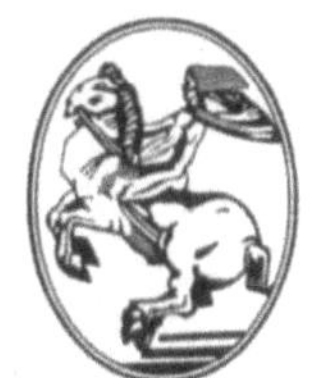

Advances and Technical Standards in Neurosurgery

Edited by

H. Krayenbühl, Zürich (Managing Editor)
J. Brihaye, Bruxelles
F. Loew, Homburg/Saar
V. Logue, London
S. Mingrino, Padova
B. Pertuiset, Paris
L. Symon, London
H. Troupp, Helsinki
M. G. Yaşargil, Zürich

Volume 4

Springer-Verlag
Wien New York 1977

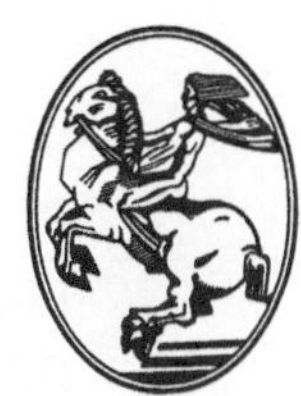

With 66 partly coloured Figures

Softcover reprint of the hardcover 1st edition 1977

Library of Congress Catalog Card Number 74-10499

ISBN-13:978-3-7091-7075-5 e-ISBN-13:978-3-7091-7073-1

DOI: 10.1007/978-3-7091-7073-1

Preface

There are two important reasons for publishing this new series entitled "Advances and Technical Standards in Neurosurgery": 1. the lack of any organized common European postgraduate training system for young neurosurgeons and 2. the language barriers, which impede the exchange of neurosurgical findings in Europe more than in other parts of the world.

The fact that the English language is well on the way to becoming the international medium at European scientific conferences is a great asset in terms of mutual understanding. Therefore the Editors have decided to publish all contributions in English, regardless of the native language of the authors.

All contributions are submitted to the entire editorial board before publication of any volume.

Our series is not intended to compete with the publications of original scientific papers in other neurosurgical journals. Our intention is, rather, to present fields of neurosurgery and related areas in which important recent advances have been made. The contributions are written by specialists in the given fields and constitute the first part of each volume.

In the second part of each volume, we publish detailed descriptions of standard operative procedures, furnished by experienced clinicians; in these articles the authors describe the techniques they employ and explain the advantages, difficulties and risks involved in the various procedures. This part is intended primarily to assist young neurosurgeons in their postgraduate training. However, we are convinced that it will also be useful to experienced, fully trained neurosurgeons.

The descriptions of standard operative procedures are a novel feature of our series, and in this it differs from the similarly entitled series "Progress in Neurological Surgery"; also, our series will be mainly, but not exclusively, a forum for European neurosurgeons. We intend as well to make available the findings of European neurosurgeons which are published in less familiar languages to neurosurgeons beyond the boundaries of the authors' countries and of Europe, and we aim to promote contacts among European neurosurgeons.

The Editors do hope that neurosurgeons throughout the world, and not only in Europe, will profit by the new series "Advances and Technical Standards in Neurosurgery".

The Editors

Contents

A. Advances

B. Technical Standards

List of Contributors

Caron, Prof. J. P., Chef du Service de Neurochirurgie, Hôpital Universitaire Henri Mondor, 51, Av. du Maréchal de Lattre-de-Tassigny, F-94010 Créteil, France.

Debrun, Prof. Dr. G., Chef du Département de Neuro-Radiologie, Hôpital Universitaire Henri Mondor, 51, Av. du Maréchal de Lattre-de-Tassigny, F-94010 Créteil, France.

Gasser, Dr. J. C., Institut für Anästhesiologie, Kantonsspital Zürich, Rämistraße 100, CH-8091 Zürich, Switzerland.

Ingvar, Prof. Dr. D. H., Department of Neurophysiology, Clinic of the University, Hospital Lund, S-22590 Lund, Sweden.

Lacour, Dr. P., Chef de Clinique Assistant, Service de Neuro-Radiologie, Hôpital Universitaire Henri Mondor, 51, Av. du Maréchal de Lattre-de-Tassigny, F-94010 Créteil, France.

Lassen, Prof. Dr. N. A., Department of Clinical Physiology, Bispebjerg Hospital, Bispebjerg Bakke 23, DK-2400 København NV, Denmark.

Lumley, J. S. P., F. R. C. S., Surgical Professorial Unit, St. Bartholomew's Hospital, London EC 1, Great Britain.

Rétif, Dr. J., Clinique Neurochirurgicale, Université Libre de Bruxelles, Rue Héger Bordet, 1, B-1000 Bruxelles, Belgium.

Smith, R. D., M.D., Barrow Neurological Institute, 350 West Thomas Road, Phoenix, AZ 85013, U.S.A.

Symon, L., T. D., F.R.C.S., Consultant Neurosurgeon, Gough Cooper Department of Neurological Surgery, The National Hospital, Queen Square, London WC1N 3BG, Great Britain.

Taylor, Prof. Dr. G. W., Surgical Professorial Unit, St. Bartholomew's Hospital, London EC1, Great Britain.

Yaşargil, Prof. Dr. M. G., Neurochirurgische Universitätsklinik, Kantonsspital Zürich, Rämistraße 100, CH-8091 Zürich, Switzerland.

A. Advances

Clinical Relevance of Cerebral Blood Flow Measurements

N. A. Lassen and D. H. Ingvar

Department of Clinical Physiology, Bispebjerg Hospital, Copenhagen (Denmark) and Department of Clinical Neurophysiology, University Hospital, Lund (Sweden)

With 2 partly coloured Figures

Contents

Introduction

In 1945 Kety in collaboration with Schmidt developed the nitrous oxide method for measuring the average cerebral blood flow (CBF) and the average cerebral metabolic rate of oxygen ($CMRO_2$) in man[1]. The method has given us a solid basis for understanding the overall blood flow and energy metabolism of the brain in health and disease[2]. Since then, several other methods have been devised including methods allowing measurement of flow in fairly small *regions* of the brain (rCBF) using radioisotopes. And now the cerebral circulation is probably better understood than that of any other organ of the body. It is then pertinent to ask, whether the rather massive clinical and experimental research on CBF has yielded a practical fall-out? This is the topic of the present paper.

We shall neglect indirect usefulness. Neuroanaesthesiology will, for example, not be considered, although this discipline is today to a large extent based on concepts and facts derived from studies of CBF and of intracranial pressure, viz. the importance of avoiding cerebral vasodilator stimuli[3, 4]. We are here solely concerned with clinical relevance in the strict sense, *i.e.*, the application of CBF measurement in clinical situations where the "cost-benefit" ratio is reasonably balanced towards a benefit for the individual studied: situations in which diagnostic, therapeutic or prognostic decisions concerning a given patient are in a decisive manner influenced by the information on CBF obtained.

I. Carotid Surgery and Other Forms of Surgical Intervention on Brain Arteries

During surgery on the carotid arteries on the neck for repair of stenosing and/or ulcerating arterio-sclerotic lesions a temporary clamping of the internal carotid artery is necessary. In this situation an adequate perfusion of the brain can be secured by the use of a temporary by-pass. But, there is good evidence that only a minority of patients, say 25%, actually need such a shunt, the majority having sufficient collaterals to keep up an adequate flow in the ipsilateral hemisphere during the clamping. For this reason, and because the bypass procedure in itself carries some risks, it is in many centers considered of clinical relevance on the operating table to determine, in which patient a shunt should be used. In other words, one must be able to monitor the adequacy of cerebral perfusion during a temporary clamping of the carotid. The conclusion reached by Sundt and coworkers is that both EEG recordings and measurement of CBF should be used for this purpose[5].

Measurement of CBF is made by the ^{133}Xenon injection method, that allows repeated measurements to be made with a time interval of about 10 minutes[6, 7]. ^{133}Xenon gas dissolved in physiological saline (about 1 mCi/ml) is injected as a bolus (about 1 ml) into the surgically exposed internal carotid artery. Immediately after arrival of the bolus in the ipsilateral middle cerebral artery territory (2–3 seconds following the injection) the internal carotid artery is clamped. The washout curve is recorded by a single scintillation detector coupled to a logarithmic ratemeter writing on a strip chart recorder as well as on an oscilloscope placed so, that the surgeon can inspect the curve immediately. The CBF is calculated in ml/100 g/min using the *initial slope*, *i.e.*, the slope over the first one minute, by the equation

$$\text{CBF} = 2 \cdot (\text{slope of curve})\ \text{ml/100 g/min}$$

where the slope is expressed in percent of a decade per minute[8]. A value of less than 20 ml/100 g/min, *i.e.*, a slope of less than 10 percent of a decade per minute, constitutes evidence of cerebral ischemia of a degree harmful to tissue nutrition. In such cases there is a need for inserting a temporary by-pass shunt[5, 9, 10].

Electroencephalography should also be used, so as to have a continuous monitoring system throughout the carotid operation[5]. The initial signs of ischemia can usually be clearly discerned, especially if the level of anaesthesia is constant. However, artifacts of movement and of other types may render it difficult to use the EEG as a sole monitor. We therefore agree with Sundt and coworkers[5], that it is best to use two independent monitoring systems, one continuous and qualitative (EEG) and one discontinuous and quantitative (CBF).

Comments: Monitoring the adequacy of cerebral perfusion by *oxygen tension* measurements on blood taken from the ipsilateral internal jugular vein or the ipsilateral transverse sinus has been abandoned: the variable, and often very large, drainage from the opposite side precludes reliable and representative results. The simple measurement of the *stump pressure*, *i.e.*, the blood pressure in the distal segment of the occluded internal carotid artery should also be considered. This mode of monitoring the safety of the temporary occlusion is widely used. Yet, Sundt and coworkers (personal communication) have found, that there is no sharp critical stump pressure level, say of 50 mmHg. Although most patients do have an adequate CBF (above 20 ml/100 g/min) and an unchanged EEG if the stump pressure is above 50 mmHg, occasionally this is not so. This observation is in consonance with the fact that patients with chronic hypertension cannot tolerate acute hypotension to the same low pressure levels as can normotensives. To use two different critical stump pressure limits, *e.g.*, 50 mmHg in normotensives and 70 mmHg in hypertensives, would not really be too safe either. It is not always possible to ascertain the habitual blood pressure level of a given patient.

Preoperative monitoring of CBF is also applicable to other forms of surgical interventions on brain vessels, such as extra-intracranial shunting procedures[11]. A special example is that of *carotid ligation* as a treatment for certain cases of intracranial aneurysms. In this situation the usefulness of peroperative CBF measurements has been well documented[12].

II. Focal Cortical Epilepsy

In patients with cortical seizures, *e.g.*, in form of fits of jerking movements of an arm or a leg, it is surprisingly often difficult to localize the focus. The clinical manifestations cannot always serve as a reliable guide, since the initiating cortical focus or "trigger zone" may lie at some distance from that part of the cortex, which gives rise to overt clinical symptoms. Furthermore, conventional neuroradiological procedures, including computerized axial tomography[13] also fail, as is even the case at autopsy, to reveal cerebral pathology in many cases. EEG, to summarize a vast amount of literature and of clinical experience, is only of limited help. Frequently there is no paroxysmal activity to be seen, sometimes not even during clinically manifest focal cortical seizure activity. And, when positive, the EEG most often fails to show a sharply localized focus.

Recent clinical studies of *regional cerebral blood flow* (*rCBF*) suggest, that this parameter can be of considerable value for localizing an epileptogenic focus[14]. Before presenting the evidence, some general remarks are pertinent. During a manifest seizure the focus is *electrically hyperactive* as well as *metabolically hyperactive.* The local blood flow in the focal region is markedly increased. Between the seizures, in the interictal phase, the focus has in many instances, in animal models as well as in man, been shown *also to be hyperactive,* albeit at a lower level and often in a more confined area. We call this state *subictal* to indicate that the trigger zone is active, but not (not quite) able to induce a clinical seizure.

There is often paroxysmal EEG activity in the interictal phase and this may be taken as further evidence of what we like to call subictal activity. We have found that rCBF is in many cases increased over an epileptogenic focus even when there are no manifest seizure symptoms or EEG abnormalities. We have concluded that such regions of focal hyperemia represent subictal epileptiform activity and better reveal the site of the focus than during manifest seizures, because then larger parts of the cortex are activated and the cortical hyperemia is more widespread.

Our series of patients with focal epilepsy comprises 10 patients all with lateralized motor, or sensori-motor seizures[14]. The patients were out-patients and had recurrent attacks difficult to control by medication. rCBF was measured by the ^{133}Xenon method, using a *Multidetector Scintillation Camera*[15] especially designed for dynamic radioisotope studies in 254 regions simultaneously. Since all 254 detectors work in parallel it follows, that two gamma rays hitting two different crystals at precisely the same time can be recorded. This is in contrast to conventional single crystal gamma cameras, in which the coincidence loss is much higher. As a consequence, the maximal counting rate of the Multidetector Scintillation Camera is 100 times greater then that of the conventional Gamma cameras. The *initial slope* as computed on the logarithmically transformed data is used for calculating rCBF. This is performed on-line on a minicomputer and the results are displayed on a TV-monitor with 16 colour levels so as to enable immediate interpretation of the data.

In all patients the EEG was performed simultaneously with the rCBF measurements. Three of the epilepsy patients were studied both during a seizure and interictally, six were only studied interictally, and one only during a seizure. The important finding was, that *in all nine patients measured* interictally we found (spontaneously or following photic stimulation) a marked localized rCBF increase in those areas, which in all likelihood constituted the origin of the seizure. In other words, the epileptogenic focus appeared to be clearly visible in all nine patients. Hence, according to the concepts outlined above, all nine patients showed that in the *subictal* stage the rCBF within the focus was changed enough to be measurable. Expressed otherwise, this means that a localized cortical mass of at least 1 cm^3 must be activated enough to change rCBF by approximately 30 percent.

The EEG, recorded during the rCBF studies showed a distinct focal abnormality in only two of the nine cases, and it was completely normal in two of them.

Case History

A 62-year-old man who two years previously had had recurrent seizures in the right-sided extremities, carotid angiography and EEG normal. Now admitted with continuous seizure activity consisting of small jerking movements (1 per sec) of right foot, consciousness unimpaired, EEG mostly normal, but on rare occasions with bilateral theta paroxysms. A carotid angiography and a Tc^{99m}-pertechnetate brain scintigraphy were normal. A computerized axial tomography of the brain showed cortical and central atrophy which was most pronounced in the left parietal region. The rCBF study was made on the third day of the continuous seizure.

rCBF study of the left side (Fig. 1): The first flow study, made during the seizure, showed a marked focal flow increase in the postcentral-parietal region. The seizure stopped after diazepam administration (2 mg in the internal carotid artery) and the subsequent flow study, made in the interictal period, showed a focal flow increase which was less pronounced but situated within the same region as that seen during the manifest seizure.

The seizure started again after 15 minutes and the two following flow studies showed a gradual change in the flow picture towards that found in the first study. Autoregulation was tested and found normal (MABP was elevated from 95 to 130 mm Hg by an *i.v.* angiotensin infusion). The EEG was completely normal during the flow studies, even when the patient had the manifest seizure.

The clinical relevance of localizing subictally active trigger zones in focal epilepsy cannot be fully evaluated as yet, as to the therapeutic and prognostic consequences. But, it appears safe to conclude that rCBF measurements in focal cortical epilepsy improves the possibility of localizing foci for surgical excision. We do not know yet, how often a detectable *subictal* state *i.e.*, a focal hyperemia is

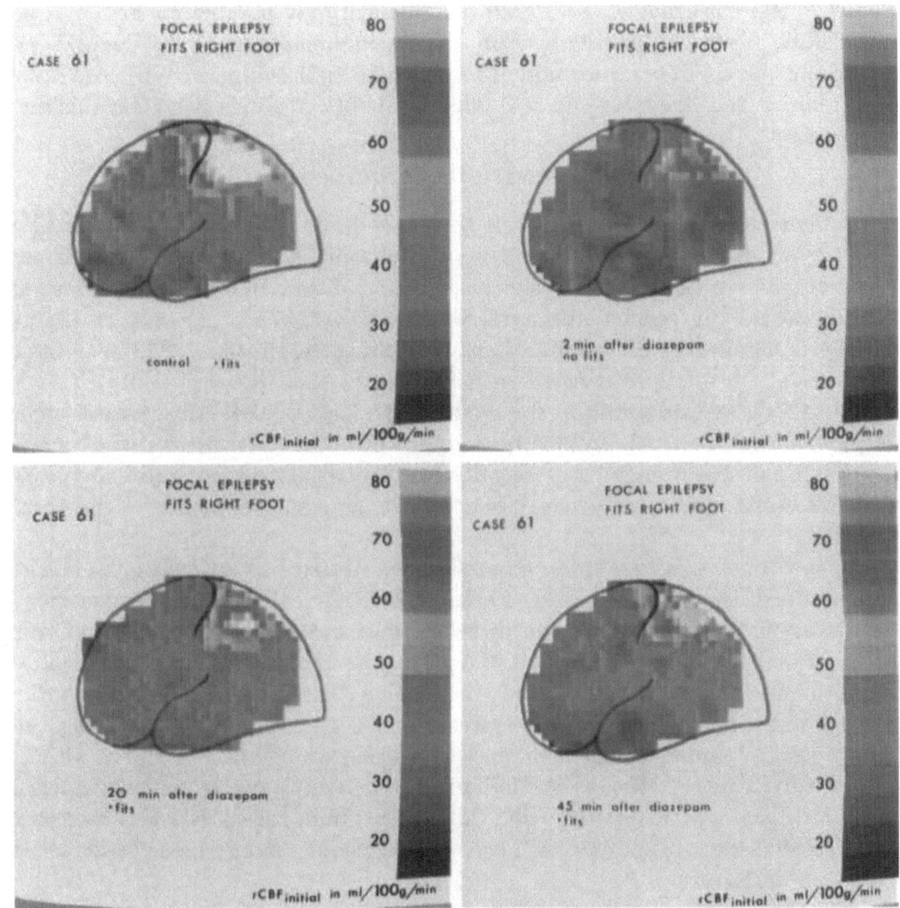

Fig. 1. Focal cortical epilepsy studied during seizure with the ^{133}Xenon intra-carotid cerebral blood flow method. rCBF is studied in 254 areas each about 1 cm^2 using a Multidetector Gamma Camera. The hyperemic epileptogenic focus is seen (upper left); Diazepam 2 mg intracarotid stops clinical seizures temporarily and markedly reduces the focus (upper right); after Diazepam seizures reappear and the focus gradually returns to its previous size. EEG shows no paroxysmal activity

present or can be provoked. It remains a possibility that all our patients by coincidence were in this phase. However, if the rCBF study proves negative, one may, like in routine EEG, provoke subictal hyperactivity, using intermittent light stimulation, hyperventilation, analeptic drugs and other provocation maneuvres.

It should be noted that the spatial resolution of the multidetector scintillation camera is limited. In the plane of the camera head it is about 1 cm (Full Width Half Maximum). But, in the depth the resolution is poor, ^{133}Xe having a half-thickness of radiation absorption of appr. 4 cm in brain tissue. Thus, superposition of many tissue layers cannot be avoided, as cannot either the difficulties in recording signals from deeper brain structures. Three-dimensional rCBF studies or measurement of local brain metabolism may become possible in a not too distant future, using the section scan techniques devised by Kuhl[16], *i.e.*, essentially the CAT-scan technique as applied to radioisotopes. With such tools a search for the epileptogenic foci may probably attain a very high clinical relevance.

III. Severe Brain Damage

Patients who have been exposed to severe brain hypoxia, brain trauma or other severe injuries sometimes end up in a chronic state of coma or semicoma. We exempt here the relatively short lasting condition of total brain infarction ("Brain death"), in which all brain structures above segment C 1 are permanently destroyed, abolishing all brain reflexes including respiration. This condition, which usually last only 3–5 days is usually diagnosed without difficulty clinically and by EEG, and, in addition by a qualitative test of CBF (four vessel angiography showing no tracer inflow inside the skull). The patients we will consider below are not brain dead: they usually breathe spontaneously and show as we shall see, some degree of arousability as well as some remaining higher brain functions.

In such cases of severe brain damage a quantitative assessment of the degree and extent of the brain injury is of considerable clinical relevance (sometimes in particular for the relatives of the patient). Measurement of cerebral blood flow (CBF and rCBF) and metabolism ($CMRO_2$) can be of distinct help in this context. Before summarizing the clinical study on which we base this contention, an outline of CBF and $CMRO_2$ in comatose states may be appropriate. It has long been known that in chronic coma the global (average of whole brain) CBF and $CMRO_2$ is markedly reduced, often to one half or even less of the values in awake normal man (50 ml/100 g/min for CBF, and 3.3 ml/100 g/min for $CMRO_2$). *The severity of the brain damage can, as we shall show, be assessed by measuring the reduction in* CBF *and* $CMRO_2$.

Our clinical series consisted of 35 patients of which 22 had suffered traumatic head injury which in 15 cases was caused by traffic accidents[17]. All patients, except one, were institutionalized. Most of them were deeply comatose, several were highly stuporous, or somnolent, eight patients showed signs of severe dementia and three of moderate dementia. The following diagnostic categories could be outlined:

1. *Complete or incomplete apallic syndromes*: Patients with diffuse and massive, more or less complete destruction of neocortical structures, without major brain stem injury. These patients showed complete loss of all higher functions, while brain stem mechanisms including respiration and some arousability appeared intact.

2. *Coma/stupor*: Patients with damage mainly to the upper brain stem (the reticular core) without signs of major focal neocortical defect. These patients were deeply comatose or stuporous, showing an absence or a very reduced arousability.

3. *Akinetic mutism, locked-in-syndromes, coma vigile*: Patients with damage to the upper pons, and/or mesial hemisphere structures. These patients showed some signs of a retained conscious perception, while their motor behaviour, including speech, was almost completely absent.

4. *Severe dementia*, usually in combination with signs of major focal neurological deficit: Patients with diffuse and/or focal neocortical damage.

5. *Moderate dementia* with limited, or no signs of focal neurological deficit: Patients with diffuse neocortical damage mainly.

Two typical cases will be described below:

Case 1: Incomplete apallic syndrome after cerebral anoxia. This patient (male 33 years) was diabetic since five years and had increasing alcohol problems with abstinence seizures. He was found deeply unconscious at home with aspiration pneumonia. Following acute resuscitation, the patient remained deeply comatose with complete loss of all higher functions and a severe depression of the EEG. The brain stem reflexes were retained with spontaneous respiration and vasomotor regulation, as well as normal corneal and pupillary reflexes. There were lively spinal reflexes and Babinski's signs bilaterally. On stimulation, the patient showed primitive movements, swallowing and respiration.

An rCBF study five months after the anoxic injury showed a markedly reduced mean flow (Fig. 2). The distribution was also highly abnormal with a lack of the "hyperfrontal" pattern pertaining to normal wakefulness. There were furthermore no changes during electrical cutaneous stimulation of the hand contralateral to the hemisphere studied. Nor was there any change of the rCBF pattern when the patient was spoken to. The patient died two weeks after the study and at autopsy a generalized, severe loss of cortical neurons was found. Some frontal and occipital cortical regions were better preserved. The cerebellum, the thalamus, the basal ganglia, and the brain stem were relatively well preserved.

This patient examplifies the rCBF findings in a chronic patient with massive neocortical injury in which there were no signs of remaining higher functions. The cerebral blood flow was reduced to a level of about 20% of the normal. The distribution of the resting flow was also abnormal and it was not possible to change the rCBF pattern by activation procedures. All these findings indicated a total loss of telencephalic structures, a conclusion, which was confirmed at autopsy.

Case 2. Akinetic mutism following head injury. This patient (male, 30 years) was hit on the right forehead by a heavy weight about 3.5 yr. prior to the rCBF study. On admission he was deeply unconscious and showed extension spasms. He was operated for a large impression fracture in the right parieto-temporal region and remained deeply unconscious for about 2.5 yr. Following this he showed feeble signs of awakening. At the time of the rCBF study the patient lay mute and motionless in his bed with signs of a spastic quadriplegia, most marked on the right side. He did not speak at all nor answer when spoken to. Some moderately coordinated eye movements were observed and he gave an impression of sometimes following objects shown to him with his gaze. The EEG showed a continuous severe slow wave abnormality with focal delta and occasional paroxysmal discharges in the right temporal region. On the left side there was a general slowing. On stimulation, arousal responses were recorded in the EEG.

Two resting rCBF determinations on the left side showed identical results. The mean flow was moderately reduced to about 80% of the normal and there was a notable lack of high flows in the frontal region (the normal "hyperfrontal" resting pattern). When the patient was shown a series of pictures and asked to look at them, a remarkably large increase of the flow was observed which was most marked in rolandic and postcentral structures, where certain detectors recorded a flow increase of more than 100%. In this case the rCBF study confirmed the presence of a high mean flow level, fully compatible with the existence of conscious perception. Activation with a simple picture test gave clear-cut evidence of cerebral reactions of a type also compatible with the assumption that the patient had perceived the content of the pictures shown. The rCBF finding was in contrast to the akinetic and mute appearance of the patient which did not change appreciably during the test.

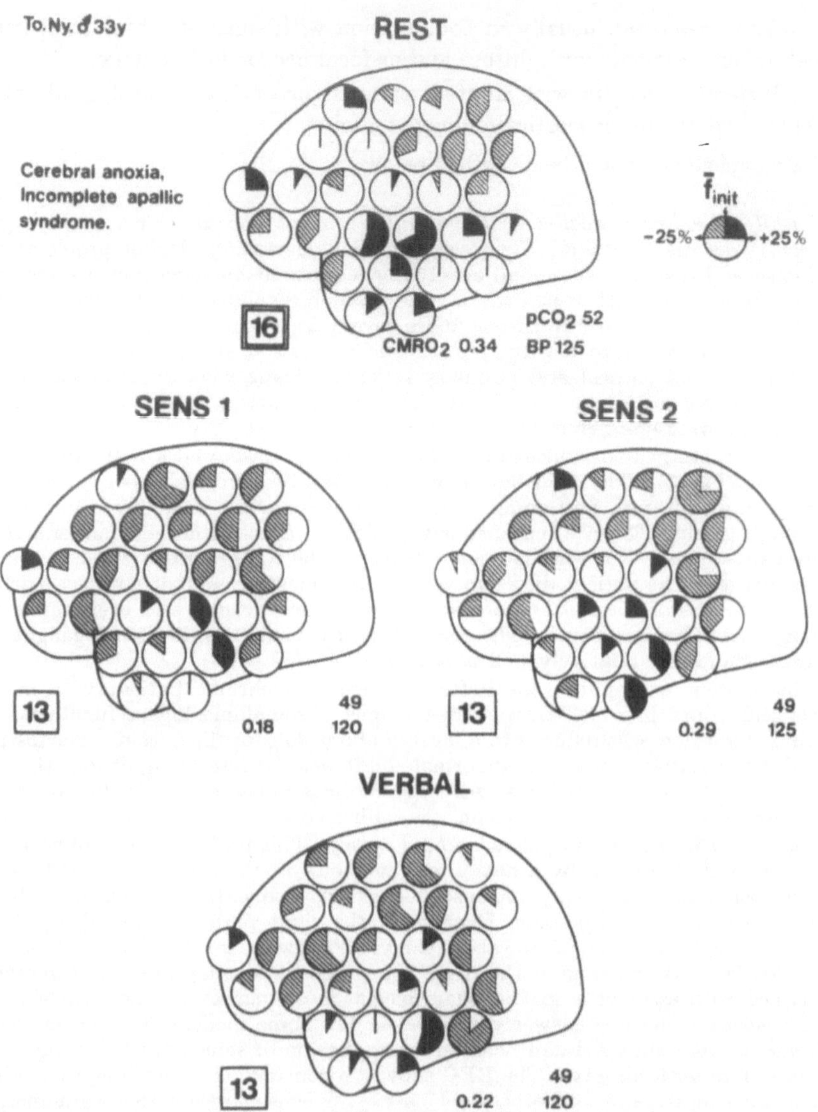

Fig. 2. Apallic syndrome studied with the [133]Xenon intracarotid injection method. rCBF is studied in 32 areas each about 6 cm^2 using 32 scintillation probes. The clock-like symbol represents the regional flow relative to the hemispheric mean value. The exceptionally low flows (about 10 ml/100 g/min in most regions) are not reacting to touch (sensory stimulation 1), to painful stimulation (sensory stimulation 2) or to loud verbal stimulation: A completely non-reactive state. The study was made with a 32-detector equipment, but only 27 detectors recorded sufficient radioactivity for flow calculations

The experience summarized above suggests that rCBF and $CMRO_2$ measurements permit one to diagnose the localization and severity of cortical dysfunction. This has contributed to a new classification of such states, a classification which may be of use as a basis for the planning of the future care of the patient. In this context the question of the state of consciousness—and ability to suffer—of the patient is central. It is imperative to establish the degree of consciousness of patients with brain lesions, and this is often difficult if the patient lacks all forms of behavioural responses to sensory stimulation. Even EEG studies are not always of decisive help, and EEG will in any event only yield qualitative evidence. It appears that by means of rCBF studies one can establish if the brain in a given patient has a functional level at which consciousness even in reduced form probably exists or not. And, by the use of stimulation tests, one may find out if normal cerebral reactions to sensory stimulation and normal CBF correlates to perceptual processing are present. To be concrete, the demonstration in a chronic patient of a very low functional state of the brain and absence of pain reactions in the brain (like in the apallic state: Case 1) justifies conservatism in therapeutic procedures. The finding of a high functional level and perceptual changes on complex stimulation—like in akinetic mutism—must, on the other hand, lead to proper therapeutic measures which take into consideration that the patient is alert and conscious, in spite of a complete lack of behavioural reactions.

Discussion

The techniques for *regional* CBF measurements have only recently reached a resolution allowing finer details to be seen. Our preliminary experience with the 254 detector instrument applied to focal cortical epilepsy illustrates this point. The possible clinical usefulness of such rCBF measurements as adjunct to cerebral angiography remains to be explored. It would seem in particular promising to make a detailed study of stroke cases, where conventional angiography so often fails to show relevant lesions. Paulsons coarse-resolution rCBF studies revealed hyperemic or ischemic brain regions in most of angiographically negative cases studied in the acute state[18]. Today a more precise description of these abnormalities is possible. It gives a means of classifying (diagnosing) apoplexy cases, that should improve our changes of developing therapeutic approaches and of predicting the clinical course. To give a specific example, we are under the impression that angiographically negative stroke cases with regional brain hyperemia ("luxury perfusion") have a rather favorable prognosis, and that in such cases hypertension should perhaps be treated more energetically than in stroke cases with ischemia.

There are other clinical conditions where rCBF measurements may be of relevance. We shall list some, that we consider promising, but yet not quite firmly established.

1. *Organic dementia*: to aid neuropsychological exploration of subsymptoms of the syndrome[19], to distinguish between the more common primary parenchymatous senile/presenile brain disease from the less common multiinfarct dementia[20], to recognize (diagnose) the pseudo-dementia state of Korsakoff's psychosis[21].
2. *Subarachnoid haemorrhage*: for assessing if an arterial aneurism is likely to bleed again serial determinations with non-traumatic CBF techniques are advocated[22].
3. *Brain death*: for demonstration of complete cessation of cerebral circulation at the bed side and hence avoiding the somewhat heroic application of four-vessel angiography in such cases; the intravenous ^{99m}Tc injection method is employed[23].

Neuropsychological exploration of the deficits resulting from various lesions. This topic, mentioned under organic dementia, has a wider scope. To give an example, the study of *aphasia* should benefit from knowledge of the normal pattern of brain cortex activation as revealed by increase in rCBF and of the alternations of this pattern in the patient. For such studies both ^{133}Xe injection and ^{133}Xe inhalation rCBF studies may be of use. Computerized axial tomography (CAT-scans) and conventional static scintigrams should be applied to the same type of exploration. But, these techniques do not to nearly the same extent as rCBF reflect the *functional* state of the brain cortex.

Conclusion

In concluding this brief review we want to add a few comments on the use of CBF studies for *screening purposes*. The semiquantitative, non-traumatic techniques (^{99m}Tc injection and ^{133}Xe inhalation combined with external counting) have been discussed in this context. This proposal is, unfortunately, based on an erroneous concept. Screening demands techniques that are highly sensitive to the abnormality looked for and yet only has a relatively low rate of false positives. We don't know of "preclinical" neurological disease states that could be revealed. We don't know the test that could be applied even if the high resolution intra-arterial rCBF technique was used completely freely: how to diagnose the patient who is going to have a stroke tomorrow? With this we have expressed our conviction that selected tests involving high resolution measurements and applied to specific clinical situations is what pays.

References

1. Kety, S. S., Schmidt, C. F., 1945: The determination of cerebral blood flow in man by the use of nitrous oxide in low concentration. Amer. J. Physiol. *143*, 53—66.
2. Lassen, N. A., 1959: Cerebral blood flow and oxygen consumption in man. Physiol. Rev. *39*, 183—238.
3. Jennett, W. B., Barker, J., Fitch, W., McDowall, D. G., 1969: Effect of anaesthesia on intracranial pressure in patients with space-occupying lesions. Lancet *1*, 61—64.
4. Alexander, S. C., Lassen, N. A., 1970: Cerebral circulatory response to acute brain disease. Implications for anesthetic practice. Anesthesiology *32*, 60—68.
5. Sundt, T. M., Sharbrough, F. W., Anderson, R. E., Michenfelder, J. D., 1974: Cerebral blood flow measurements and electroencephalograms during carotid endarterectomy. J. Neurosurg. *41*, 310—320.
6. Lassen, N. A., Ingvar, D. H., 1963: Regional cerebral blood flow measurement in man. A review. Arch. Neurol. *9*, 615—622.
7. Høedt-Rasmussen, K., Sveinsdottir, E., Lassen, N. A., 1966: Regional cerebral blood flow in man determined by intra-arterial injection of radioactive inert gas. Circulat. Res. *18*, 237—247.
8. Olesen, J., Paulson, O. B., Lassen, N. A., 1971: Regional cerebral blood flow in man determined by the initial slope of the clearance of intra-arterially injected ^{133}Xe. Stroke *2*, 519—540.
9. Trojaborg, W., Boysen, G., 1973: Relation between EEG, regional cerebral blood flow and internal carotid artery pressure during carotid endarterectomy. Electroenceph. clin. Neurophysiol. *34*, 61—69.
10. Boysen, G., 1973: Cerebral hemodynamics in carotid surgery. Acta neurol. scand. *49*, suppl. 59.
11. Schmiedek, P., Steinhoff, H., Gratzl, O., Şteude, U., Enzenbach, R., 1972: rCBF-measurements in patients treated for cerebral ischemia by extra-intracranial vascular anastomosis. Europ. Neurol. *6*, 364—368.
12. Jennet, W. B., Harper, A. M., Gillespie, F. C., 1966: Measurement of regional cerebral blood-flow during carotid ligation. Lancet *2*, 1162—1163.

13. Bogdanoff, B. M., Stafford, C. R., Green, L., Gonzalez, C. F., 1975: Computerized transaxial tomography in the evaluation of patients with focal epilepsy. Neurology *25*, 1013—1017.
14. Hougaard, K., Oikawa, T., Sveinsdottir, E., Skinhøj, E., Ingvar, D. H., Lassen, N. A., 1976: Regional cerebral blood flow in patients with focal cortical epilepsy. Arch. Neurol. *33*, 527—542.
15. Sveinsdottir, E., Larsen, B., Rommer, P., Lassen, N. A.: A multidetector scintillation camera with 254 channels. J. Nucl. Med. (in press).
16. Kuhl, D. E., Edwards, R. Q., 1968: Reorganizing data from transverse section scans using digital processing. Radiology *91*, 975—983.
17. Ingvar, D. H., Cerea, M. Gadea, 1975: Assessment of severe damage to the brain by multi-regional measurement of cerebral blood flow. In: "Outcome of Severe Damage to the Central Nervous System", Ciba Symposium, p. 97—120. Amsterdam: Elsevier Publ.
18. Paulson, O. B., Lassen, N. A., Skinhøj, E., 1970: Regional cerebral blood flow in apoplexy without arterial occlusion. Neurology (Minneap.) *20*, 125—138.
19. Hagberg, B., Ingvar, D. H., 1976: Cognitive reduction in prenile dementia related to regional abnormalities of the cerebral blood flow. Brit. J. Psychiat. *128*, 209—222.
20. Hachinski, V. C., Iliff, Linette D., Zilkha, E., du Boulay, G. H., McAllister, V. L., Marshall, J., Ross Russell, R. W., Symon, L., 1975: Cerebral blood flow in dementia. Arch. Neurol. *32*, 632—637.
21. Hachinski, V. V., Lassen, N. A., Marshall, J., 1974: Multi-infarct dementia. A cause of mental deterioration in the elderly. Lancet *2*, 207—209.
22. Taylor, A. R., Kak, V. K., 1966: Cerebral blood flow in subarachnoid hemorrhage. In "Research on the Cerebral Circulation", III. Int. Salzburg Conference, 364—375.
23. Korein, J., Braunstein, P., Kricheff, I., Lieberman, A., Chase, N., 1975: Radioisotopic technique as a test to detect circulatory deficit associated with cerebral death. Circulation *51*, 924—939.

Extra-Cranial Surgery for Cerebrovascular Disease

G. W. Taylor and J. S. P. Lumley

Surgical Professorial Unit, St. Bartholomew's Hospital, London E.C. 1 (Great Britain)

With 6 Figures

Contents

The crippling effect of a completed stroke, not only on the patient, but also on all his associates is undeniable and any means of preventing such an occurrence must receive the closest possible attention.

It is now over twenty years since the first reports appeared of prophylactic vascular surgery for patients with stroke syndrome. During this period a considerable literature has appeared on the subject and it is perhaps now pertinent to consider the merits of these surgical procedures.

This review will firstly survey the factors leading up to the development of this form of surgery and continue by discussing the mechanism of the transient ischaemic attack (TIA) and the aetiology and clinical features of the stroke syndrome. Further sections will consider the selection of patients for surgery, the surgical procedures involved and the results of surgery in these patients.

Development of Surgery for Strokes

When following the development of this surgical field two factors of paramount importance emerge, a) the realisation that many strokes result from disease of the extra-cranial vessels and b) the fact that major strokes are often preceded by TIA's.

The relationship between cerebral function and the extra-cranial vessels is reflected in the Greek derivation of the word "carotid" which literally means "to stupify" or "to plunge into deep sleep". The pathological relationship was emphasised by Abercrombie (1828) when he likened cerebral infarction to limb gangrene, when the limb's blood supply was compromised. In 1844 Todd described a stroke in a patient with a dissecting aneurysm of the innominate artery and Virchow (1856) reported similar effects in patients with thrombosis of the carotid bifurcation. Savory (1856) was probably the first to record occlusive disease affecting the aortic arch and in 1875 the clinical features relating to obstructive aortic arch disease were detailed by Broadbent. Gowers (1875) described cerebral symptoms and the eventual death of a patient with left atrial disease and was able to demonstrate, at post mortem, that these symptoms were embolic in origin. Chiari (1905) in a classical but much neglected paper noted that "endarteriitis chronica deformans" preferentially affected the carotid arteries. He also found that cerebral embolism originated from atheroma in the carotid bifurcation. Hunt (1914) from his clinical studies noted that transient ischaemic attacks often preceded a major stroke, but it was not until Fisher's work (1951, 1954) that the relevance of these findings to possible surgical intervention was considered.

In the early 1950's, two important papers were published on carotid artery surgery. The first was by Strully *et al.* in 1953. These workers reported an unsuccessful operation on the carotid vessels in a stroke patient. In the following year Eastcott, Pickering and Rob reported the first successful reconstructive procedure in this group of patients and, although two successful procedures had gone unreported prior to that date (Carrea *et al.* 1955, Thompson 1973 a), this paper has had a lasting influence on the subsequent development of surgery for this condition. The first reported endarterectomy, the present procedure of choice was described by Cooley *et al.* in 1956.

The development of surgery for the vertebral arteries and the vessels arising from the aortic arch are discussed in a later section.

Mechanism of the TIA

The stroke syndrome can be classified into three categories, transient, developing and completed. In transient strokes the neurological defect is short lived and the patient is normal between attacks, whereas in a completed stroke some permanent neurological deficit remains. In the context of extra-cranial arterial disease the transient stroke is the chief indication for surgical treatment (vide infra) and the mechanism of the TIA deserves further consideration.

It is now generally agreed that there are two possible factors causing a TIA. These are, a) a temporary reduction of blood flow to the relevant cerebral area and, b) obstruction of the cerebral micro-circulation by a small embolus which subsequently disperses.

An earlier theory that TIA's could be explained by arterial spasm (Moniz *et al.* 1937) was rejected by Pickering (1948), since these symptoms are frequently retinal in origin and the retinal arteries are among the least responsive in the body.

a) *Reduction in Blood Flow.* This theory originally held pride of place because of the known high incidence of stroke following carotid ligation. This operation was first performed by Abernethy (1798) in a patient who had been gored by a cow (Hamby 1952) and was subsequently frequently undertaken for the treatment of intra-cranial aneurysms. The stroke rate following this procedure was of the order of 30% and in these instances the stroke was, of course, permanent. The relationship of blood flow reduction to the transient attack was ingeniously explained by Denny-Brown (1951) who propounded the theory of "haemodynamic crisis". This was based on the assumption that in a patient with an extra-cranial arterial stenosis sudden lowering of the blood pressure would render the stenosis "critical" and a significant fall in blood flow through the artery would occur. When the blood pressure returned to normal levels, flow improved and the neurological signs would disappear. In support of this theory Denny-Brown and Meyer (1957) were able to produce a TIA by lowering and subsequently raising the blood pressure in an animal with a localised cerebral artery stenosis.

In clinical practice, however, Alajouanine *et al.* (1960) were unable to demonstrate changes in systolic blood pressure in patients during ischaemic attacks and Kendell and Marshall (1963) failed to produce neurological symptoms by lowering the blood pressure in patients with a history of TIA's. Brice, Dowsett and Lowe (1964) demonstrated that the lumen of the internal carotid artery could be reduced by as much as 90% without interference to cerebral blood flow. This was, however, influenced by the rate of onset of the stenosis and the presence of multiple stenoses. Russell and Cranston (1961) reported that TIA's were rare after carotid ligation. The weight of opinion thus moved to favour the micro-embolisation theory.

b) *Micro-Embolisation.* The embolic theory was first suggested by Millikan *et al.* (1955) who postulated that small thrombi or cholesterol aggregations might be liberated from a localised patch of atheroma in the carotid area and cause temporary obstruction of the micro-circulation of the retina or brain. Credence was lent to this theory by the observations of Fisher (1959) who by ophthalmoscopic examination noted the presence of retinal emboli in patients undergoing TIA's. Kollarits *et al.* (1972) performed carotid angiography in 45 patients with transient attacks of visual disturbance and found a possible embolic source in the carotid vessels in 43 (96%). It is certainly true that in many of the patients with TIA's, the carotid lesion is an ulcerated plaque of atheroma with little significant stenosis (Fig. 1).

It seems likely, therefore, that the majority of TIA's are due to embolisation but the haemodynamic aspect should not be totally discounted. Reivich *et al.* (1961) in describing the subclavian steal syndrome, reported cerebral symptoms occurring during upper limb exercise, blood being diverted from the brain to the arm via the vertebral artery. Per-operative measurement of carotid blood pressure distal to a clamp site has shown that strokes are more likely to occur during clamping if the "stump pressure" is less than 25 mmHg (Moore and Hall 1969). Jennett *et al.* (1966) found that in patients with intra-cerebral aneurysms, focal symptoms followed carotid ligation if the overall cerebral blood flow was reduced by more than 25% during temporary carotid clamping. It is possible, therefore, that the flow factor may be responsible for TIA's in a small proportion of patients with carotid stenosis. The transient neurological phenomena would then presumably correspond to a period of temporary reduction in cardiac output with

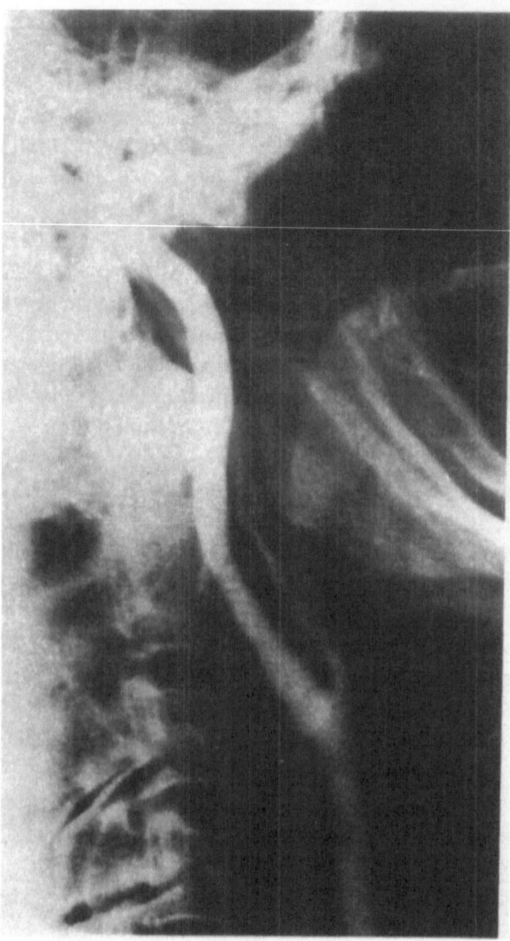

Fig. 1. Right carotid arteriogram of a **64** year old male patient presenting with contralateral TIA's. Slight irregularity of the origin of the internal carotid artery is present

consequent significant reduction of flow through the narrowed carotid artery (Fig. 2).

The collateral circulation becomes important in this context and accessory blood flow may occur between the external carotid and the ophthalmic artery, the meningeal and cerebral arteries, the occipital and vertebral arteries, the cervical and vertebral arteries and the occasionally encountered rete mirabile of the internal carotid artery. A persistent hypoglossal artery may occasionally occur and cerebral ischaemia secondary to disease of this vessel has been reported by Sutherland and Donaldson (1972). The final pathway of the collateral circulation is, however, the Circle of Willis, and anatomical variation of this important anastomotic ring is not uncommon (Alpers *et al.* 1959).

The pattern of the Circle of Willis can be recognised in the foetus from the second month of intrauterine life and the size of its contributing branches are determined by subsequent cerebral development. Paget (1944) listed the common

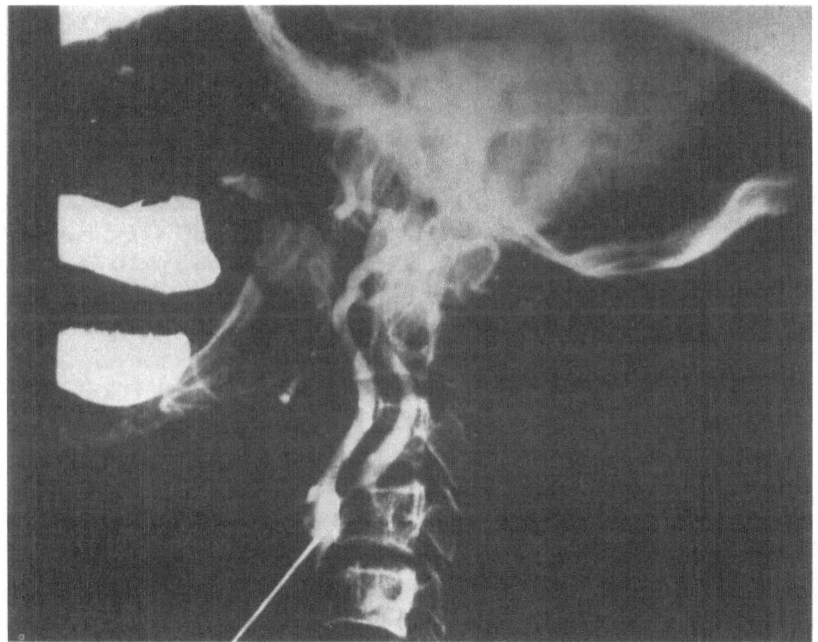

Fig. 2. Left carotid arteriogram of a 54 year old male patient presenting with contralateral TIA's. Marked stenosis of internal carotid artery origin is present

variations of the Circle of Willis as a) unequal posterior communicating arteries b) absent posterior communicating arteries and c) separate circulations to the two hemispheres, although Hamby (1952) in reviewing this field indicates diversity of opinion in the findings of different investigators. Such variation of the distribution of a cerebral vessel will obviously markedly influence the effect of extracerebral vascular disease.

Surgery may improve collateral flow and Connolly and Stemmer (1973) have reported benefit in patients with irreversibly occluded internal carotid arteries following correction of concomitant stenosis of the external carotid origin.

Aetiology of the Stroke Syndrome

In the large majority of patients, the aetiology of the stroke syndrome is atherosclerosis. This was confirmed in an arteriographic series from the Mayo Clinic (Houser and Baker 1968) in which only 28 patients of 5,000 were suffering from non-atheromatous disease. In over half of these patients, the disease is situated at the carotid bifurcation. Other sites in decreasing order of frequency are the vertebral arteries, the subclavian artery, the external carotid arteries, the innominate artery, the right subclavian artery, and the left common carotid artery. Other lesions occasionally responsible for neurological symptoms include: aneurysms of the brachio-cephalic system, these being post-traumatic, mycotic, syphilitic, post-radiotherapy and dissecting aneurysms, as well as atherosclerotic. Occasionally congenital or acquired arterio-venous fistulae, congenital malformations, kinks, coils and bands occur in the carotid region and these together with vascular trauma may give rise to neurological problems. A rare group of arterial conditions which have been sporadically recorded as requiring surgical treatment include fibro-muscular hyperplasia, medial wall necrosis, diffuse arteritis, giant cell arteritis, scleroderma, drug induced stenoses and adjacent inflammatory cervical nodes. Tumours in the region of the carotid bifurcation, *e.g.*, carotid body tumours, may give rise to neurological symptoms. All cranial and extra-cranial vessels may be affected by extra-vascular factors such as hypercoagulability states and severe hypertension. Conditions giving rise to thrombosis include pregnancy, the pill, idiopathic thrombocytopenia, polycythaemia, sickle cell anaemia, anoxia, anaemia and congestive cardiac failure. It is probable that focal neurological sequelae following severe hypotension, such as in cardiac arrest, cardiac dysrhythmia and extensive trauma only occur in patients with pre-existing asymptomatic arterial lesions.

Clinical Features of the Stroke Syndrome

Symptoms

a) Carotid Disease

TIA's in the carotid distribution are usually focal in nature with paraesthesiae or weakness of one or both contralateral limbs and classically ipsilateral visual disturbance. If the dominant hemisphere is involved dysphasia will accompany the other symptoms. Visual symptoms are present in about 40% of patients and are the sole disturbance in approximately 15% of carotid TIA's. The degree of visual defect may range from mild blurring to significant, but temporary field loss (amaurosis fugax). Headache frequently accompanies a TIA and, after multiple episodes, patients may notice impairment of memory and concentration. TIA's are usually repetitive, but their frequency can range from multiple daily disturbances to isolated episodes many months apart. The duration of the individual attack can vary from a few minutes to several hours and rarely the neurological defect may persist for 24 hours. The degree of neurological damage sustained in a completed stroke is related to the rate of onset, the duration and extent of the ischaemia and the area of brain involved. A major stroke may be accompanied by a period of unconsciousness and recovery of function, if it occurs at all, is slow and often unpredictable.

b) Vertebro-Basilar Disease

Ischaemic episodes in the vertebro-basilar territory may overlap those of the carotid distribution but they are usually less well defined. Occular symptoms tend to be more prominent and are often bilateral, they may include optic atrophy and cataract formation. Attacks of giddiness are common and motor symptoms may be bilateral in distribution. Because ocular symptoms are frequent many reports on the condition have come from ophthalmologists. The best known of these was a report from Takayasu (1908) who described absence of upper limb pulses in a young woman with bilateral cataracts. Disease of the origins of the great vessels from the aortic arch is consequently often referred to as Takayasu's disease (Caccamise and Whitman 1952). Other synonyms for this syndrome are Martorell's disease (Martorell and Fabré 1944), pulseless disease (Shimizu and Sano 1951) and perhaps the most satisfactory term—the Aortic Arch Syndrome (Frøvig 1946). The monograph of the latter author provides an important review of the subject to that time.

In patients with severe stenosis of the proximal subclavian artery, arm claudication may accompany vertebro-basilar neurological symptoms due to reversal of blood flow in the vertebral artery. This constitutes the subclavian steal syndrome described by Contorni in 1960 and so named by Reivich (1961).

Physical Signs

In between episodes the patient with TIA's will show no neurological abnormality. In carotid disease a bruit over the carotid bifurcation is present in about 66% of patients. David *et al.* (1973) reported the angiographic findings in 417 patients with a carotid bruit. In 28% of these the carotids were normal radiologically. These workers concluded that a bruit had no clear relationship to the patient's symptoms or to the angiographic findings. A possible exception to this conclusion is the presence of a characteristic high pitched bruit which usually indicates a severe degree of arterial stenosis. Sudden loss of a previously noted high pitch bruit (after, for instance, arteriography) implies complete occlusion of the artery and may call for urgent exploration of the lesion.

Investigation

In the pre-operative evaluation of the extra-cranial arterial disease arteriography plays the major role. It carries with it, however, the need for experienced personnel, elaborate instrumentation and has a small but definite morbidity and mortality risk to the patient. Consequently although it is an essential pre-operative investigation, it must be considered an unsatisfactory screening procedure. In view of this a number of non-invasive investigations have been introduced in an attempt to detect patients with possible internal carotid artery disease and also to some extent provide additional information on cerebral blood flow and the development of collaterals. One of the early investigations was that of ocular dynamometry (Svien and Hollenhorst 1956). The pressure device applied to the eye ball in this technique, however, is not without discomfort to the patient and tends to distort the globe and obliterate the curves being evaluated. The technique of oculo-plethysmography (Kartchner *et al.* 1973) provides a more sensitive measurement of arterial pressure curves. Kartchner and his colleagues suggested that bilateral ocular pulses should be recorded simultaneously, since they considered the relative timing of the two tracings was more important than absolute measurements of amplitude. These authors advised combination of this test with carotid phonangiography, the latter consisting of audio-visual analysis of cervical carotid bruit recordings, the composite diagnostic accuracy of the two tests being 91% and 86% respectively in relation to arteriographic evaluation.

The Doppler ophthalmic test (Brockenbrough 1970) was introduced to assess collateral flow through the external carotid artery in the presence of internal carotid artery disease. On compression of the superficial temporal artery in the normal person an augmentation of the supra-orbital flow can be detected by a Doppler probe. A range from augmentation to loss of flow can be noted, this being related to the degree of occlusion in the ipsilateral internal carotid artery. The directional Doppler also enables reversal of flow in this vessel to be distinguished. The Doppler ophthalmic test has been studied extensively by Machleder and Barker (Machleder and Barker 1972, Machleder 1973). Care must be taken to avoid false positive results from listening over the lateral nasal artery—false positive and false negative results are unfortunately frequent. A negative Doppler test in the presence of an internal carotid artery stenosis suggests that restoration of blood flow via the homolateral external carotid artery is minimal.

Another disadvantage of these methods is that, while providing information on internal carotid artery stenosis and occlusion, they do not detect the equally important sites of ulceration and embolisation. These methods should not, therefore, be the sole form of evaluation in the symptomatic patient. A more sophisticated form of Doppler scanning has been introduced by Thomas *et al.* (1974) for mapping of the carotid bifurcation. This demonstrates by non-invasive techniques, changes such as calcification, stenosis, irregularity, kinking and flow patterns within the internal carotid artery.

Non-invasive techniques are useful in complementing angiographic studies and may be particularly valuble in assessing the post-operative patient and following up the natural history of the disease. They add a haemodynamic dimension to the angiographic assessment and they may demonstrate previously unsuspected carotid artery disease.

In the diagnosis of extra-cranial vascular disease it is essential to obtain biplane angiography of both carotid bifurcations. The most satisfactory pictures are usually obtained by the direct carotid stab technique, the intra-cerebral blood vessels being demonstrated simultaneously and the possibility of overlooking an intra-cerebral lesion diminished. This technique has the disadvantage of not demonstrating the branches of the aortic arch and the vertebral artery origins and, if symptoms suggestive of disease at these sites are present, additional arch aortography should be undertaken, preferably via the trans-femoral route. It is possible that techniques will develop by which adequate carotid bifurcation views and intra-cerebral vascular delineation can be obtained by selective injection through the trans-femoral approach, but at present, schools differ in their approach to this problem.

There is generally good correlation in the interpretation of carotid bifurcation disease by the surgeon and the radiologist, particularly in advanced and roughened lesions (Gomensoro *et al.* 1973). The radiological diagnosis of ulceration should be suspected in the presence of penetrating niches, an irregular silhouette, the delayed washout of a medium in a segment of artery between areas of stenosis and well circumscribed double density of contrast medium superimposed on the artery (Blaisdell *et al.* 1974).

Natural History of the Atherosclerotic Lesion

In a study of a community of 2,445 people over the age of 40 years, Karp and his colleagues (1973) found 28 patients with TIA's. The incidence of this syndrome in the white population was 15.9/1000 in males and 11.5/1000 in females. A considerably higher incidence of stroke syndrome is found in patients with established arterial disease in other sites and Javid *et al.* (1974) reported an incidence of 15% in patients presenting to their vascular service with non-cerebral peripheral arterial symptoms.

Acheson and Hutchinson (1971) studied the long term outcome in 500 patients with focal cerebral vascular disease. 349 patients had established neurological defects and 53% of these worsened during the period of observation. 151 of the patients had TIA's and, of these, 62% developed a completed stroke within 4½ years. A similar study was reported by Siekert (1970) who found a 20–25% incidence of major stroke in patients with TIA's followed over a 4 year period. In all reported series carotid disease has a considerably worse prognosis than vertebro-basilar. The results of these studies emphasise the considerable risk of patients with TIA's progressing to a major stroke.

Another group of patients which has received much attention with relation to possible carotid endarterectomy has been the patient with the asymptomatic carotid bruit, this being a not infrequent finding in any vascular clinic. The natural history of this group of patients was studied by Javid *et al.* (1970) and Thompson and Patman (1970). Javid and his colleagues found that in a long term study of 145 such patients, 11 died of a stroke, 7 died of a cardiac cause and another 7 died of unrelated causes. In 93 patients undergoing a repeat angiogram, significant changes had taken place in 51 patients and 22 of these required carotid endarterectomy. The rate of atheromatous change appeared to be directly related to hypertension, to the development of cerebral symptoms, to change in the intensity of the carotid bruit and to the degree of the original stenosis.

Selection of Patients for Surgery

Of the three categories of stroke (vide supra) it is the TIA patient who benefits from surgical treatment of the extra-cranial arterial lesion. Patients with a developing stroke should not be treated surgically. Operation at this stage carries a high mortality and morbidity, from cerebral oedema secondary to revascularisation in the presence of a recent infarct. If the developing stroke concludes with a partial neurological deficit, operation can then be considered as a prophylactic measure against further extension of the stroke process. In these patients angiography and surgery should be postponed for 3–4 weeks to allow the initial infarct to mature. A proportion of these patients will show total occlusion of the relevant internal carotid artery and attempts to re-open the vessel are rarely successful and generally unwise. A not infrequent problem is total occlusion of the appropriate internal carotid with significant stenosis of the opposite vessel. In this group endarterectomy of the opposite "inappropriate" artery is a useful prophylactic manœuvre.

Thompson and Patman (1970) also advocated routine angiographic study of patients with a carotid bruit and carotid endarterectomy in asymptomatic patients with a high grade internal carotid artery stenosis. Synchronous carotid endarterectomy in patients with an asymptomatic high grade stenosis undergoing surgical treatment of abdominal aortic aneurysms or coronary artery disease was recommended by Javid *et al.* (1974).

Patients with a dense completed hemiplegia rarely improve after carotid surgery and these patients are best managed conservatively with a programme of rehabilitation.

The value of anticoagulants in TIA's has been extensively studied by Marshall (1969). These should be used in patients with a tight stenosis awaiting surgery or when the patient is unsuitable for surgery, the lesion being inaccessible or the patient's general condition being unsatisfactory.

Surgical Treatment

Anaesthesia

Anaesthetic techniques in potential stroke patients have varied considerably and there is still no universally accepted method. Initially operations were undertaken under local anaesthesia in order to monitor the patient's neurological function during a trial period of carotid clamping. In the advent of neurological deterioration general anaesthesia was rapidly induced and the patient surface cooled to 32–30 °C. A paper by Wells *et al.* in 1963 advocated routine general anaesthesia, hypercarbia and induced hypertension.

In the normal brain the circulation is related to the local metabolic requirements, carbon dioxide playing an important role in the regulatory mechanism (Kety and Schmidt 1948, Patterson *et al.* 1955). The CO_2 responsiveness of damaged brain was questioned, however, by Brawley *et al.* in 1967, these workers considering that hypercarbia could increase the cerebral blood flow to the normal tissue but at the expense of any damaged areas producing the so-called intracerebral steal. It could thus be postulated that induced hypocarbia would protect damaged tissue by the so-called "Robin Hood" effect (Lassen and Pálvölgyi 1968), blood being stolen from normal brain and increasing the blood supply to the damaged areas. Whatever technique is used adequate oxygenation is essential and every effort should be made to maintain a stable circulatory system, for auto-regulation of the cerebral blood flow is lost if the systolic blood pressure falls below 60–80 mm of Hg. Controlled ventilation is advised.

Although general anaesthesia is generally used there are still some centres who advocate continued use of regional anaesthesia (Hobson *et al.* 1974), whereas Conolly (1973) advocated the combination of neurolept analgesia and regional anaesthesia. The latter technique enables continuous direct monitoring of the patient's cerebral state, this being more sensitive than EEG recordings or cerebral blood flow measurements. In all instances continuous blood gas analysis and intra-arterial monitoring of blood pressure are desirable.

Carotid Endarterectomy

The patient is placed supine with enough head up inclination to empty the cervical venous plexuses. The neck is slightly extended and the head rotated away from the operative side. A head towel is used but the appropriate ear is left exposed to be folded forward under an adhesive drape. With a high carotid bifurcation, or with disease extending well distally in the internal carotid, the incision paralleling the anterior border of the sterno-mastoid is taken superiorly to the mastoid process. A more transverse cervical incision may be used if the arteriogram demonstrates a low carotid bifurcation. Small cutaneous branches of the cervical plexus require division but the greater occipital nerve can usually be mobilised and spared. The common facial vein and occasionally the omohyoid muscle are divided to expose the common carotid artery and its bifurcation. The hypoglossal nerve is encountered superiorly in close relationship to the carotid vessels and may need to be gently mobilised by division of a branch of the occipital artery that tethers it postero-medially. The vagus nerve is frequently applied intimately to the posterior aspect of the internal carotid artery and may be inadvertently included in an arterial occlusive clamp. Temporary recurrent laryngeal nerve palsy may follow such a mishap. Mobilisation of the carotid vessels is best done by sharp dissection and with minimal disturbance in order to avoid embolisation from the area of carotid disease. If obvious thrombus is seen on the pre-operative arteriogram the distal internal carotid artery should be clamped before the bifurcation is mobilised.

Diverse views exist as to the necessity of an intraluminal shunt during carotid endarterectomy. There are currently three schools of thought:—

a) Shunting Is Unnecessary

The "no shunt" surgeons believe that per-operative strokes are due solely to embolisation occurring during the arterial mobilisation and that occlusion of the carotid blood flow is relatively unimportant (Moore *et al.* 1973). Moreover the placement of a shunt may initiate embolism and its presence is technically restricting. Kenyon *et al.* (1972) advises large doses of heparin (3 mg/Kg) during cross-clamping, no shunt and neutralisation of the heparin at the completion of the endarterectomy.

b) Shunting Should Be Used Routinely

Protagonists of the intraluminal shunt (Javid *et al.* 1974, Thompson 1973 a) believe that it is important to maintain perfusion through the carotid and that the placement of an intraluminal shunt allows the surgeon to work in a meticulous and unhurried fashion.

c) Shunting Should Be Used Only in Selected Cases

This School advises placement of an intraluminal shunt when intra-operative measurement demonstrates poor collateral flow after carotid cross-clamping. Methods of assessment range from simple visual estimation of the back bleed from the internal carotid (Young *et al.* 1969) to sophisticated techniques for estimation of cerebral blood flow after carotid clamping (Boysen 1971, Trojaborg and Boysen 1973). The most widely used method is measurement of the blood pressure within the internal carotid distal to the point of cross-clamping. Unfortunately there is lack of agreement of the minimum level of "stump pressure" which will permit an operation to proceed safely without the use of a shunt. Moore and Hall (1969) considered a pressure of 25 mmHg acceptable, Hayes *et al.* (1972) 50 mmHg and Hobson *et al.* (1974) a level of 60 mmHg. Wylie (1974) reported on 300 patients in whom shunting was only undertaken when the stump pressure

Table 1. *Operative Mortality and Severe Stroke Morbidity in Patients Undergoing Surgery for Stroke Symptoms.* The results of Javid *et al.* (1974) include all forms of reconstructive surgery, the remainder relate to carotid endarterectomy

Without shunt	% operative mortality	and severe stroke morbidity
Bloodwell *et al.* (1968) 347 patients, TIA's and completed strokes	5.6	4.8
Bloodwell *et al.* (1968) 191 patients with TIA's	4.3	2.6
Young *et al.* (1969) 137 patients with TIA's and asymptomatic patients	4.4	2.9
De Weese *et al.* (1973) 103 patients with TIA's	1.0	5.0
With shunt		
Thompson (1973 b) 537 patients with TIA's	0.7	1.5
Javid *et al.* (1974) 1,400 patients, all groups of symptoms	2.0	1.5

was less than 50 mmHg. With this criteria shunting was required in 20% of the patients and only one mild neurological deficit resulted. Further evidence on stump pressure has come from the neurosurgical field where carotid ligation is sometimes done for intra-cranial aneurysms. Wright and Sweet (1962) considered 50 mmHg as the minimum safe level while Leech *et al.* (1974) reported that carotid ligation could be undertaken safely with a stump pressure of 60 mmHg or greater. Machleder and Barker (1974) studied stump pressure in a group of patients in which an external carotid to common carotid bypass had been inserted during internal carotid endarterectomy. They noted an average increase in back pressure of 20.9% in this group of patients.

Other workers have measured jugular venous oxygen tension (White *et al.* 1967) and EEG monitoring (Perez-Borja and Meyer 1965).

A comparison of published results from centres never using shunts and those always using them is shown in Table 1. It is our own practice to use an intraluminal shunt routinely. The Javid Shunt (Figs. 3 and 4) is an excellent device

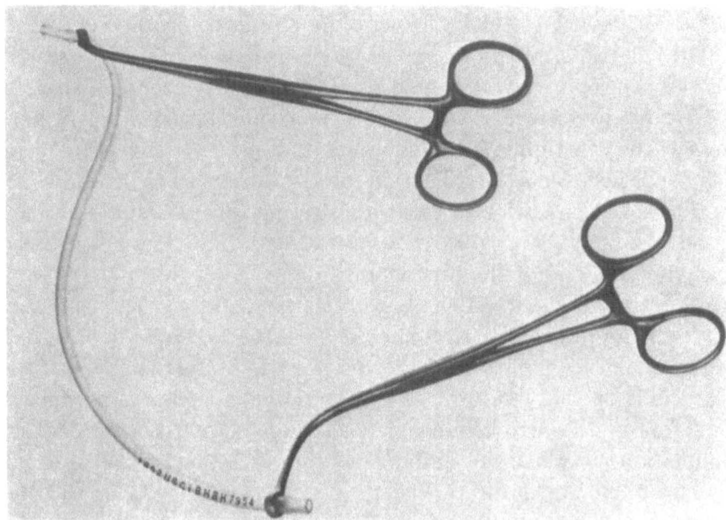

Fig. 3. Javid shunt and associated ring clamps

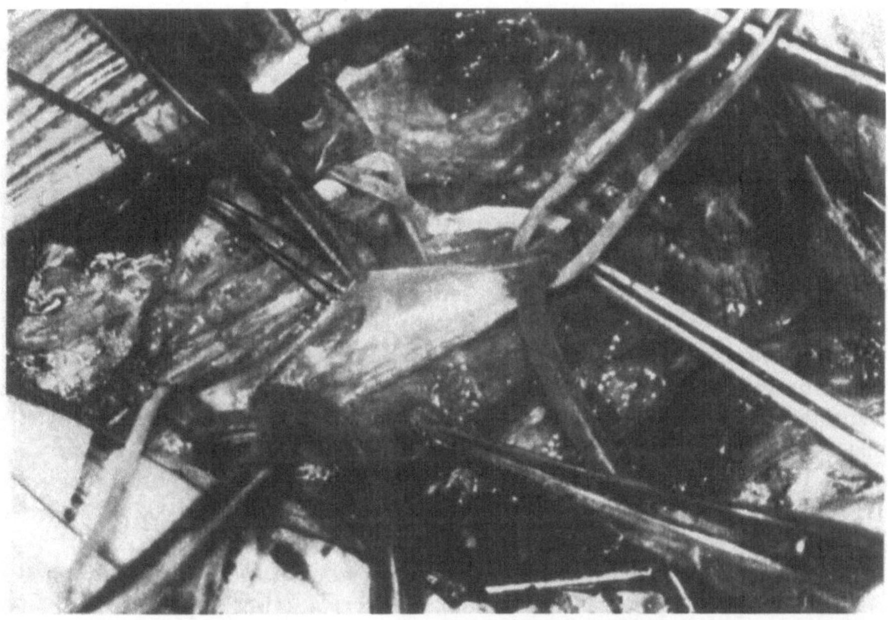

Fig. 4. Operative photograph of a left carotid endarterectomy. The arteriotomy extends into the common and internal carotid arteries. A Javid shunt is in place, note the smooth adherent line of attachment of the distal intima

for this purpose. Constructed of flexible sialastic it has a tapered bore which allows for the discrepancy in size between the common carotid and internal carotid arteries. Special ring clamps applied around the arteries hold the shunt securely in place. The proximal end is inserted into the common carotid artery first and blood allowed to flush through the shunt before and internal carotid is cannulated. This allows the escape of any fibrinous material which may have formed in the common carotid artery particularly if a carotid stab arteriogram has been recently performed. Once locked in position with the ring clamps the shunt may be safely manipulated to allow adequate access for the endarterectomy, and is removed just before completion of the arteriotomy closure. Systemic heparinisation is advised prior to carotid clamping regardless of whether a shunt is being used. An intravenous dose of 5,000–10,000 units does not usually require neutralisation at the end of the procedure.

The arteriotomy is made on the antero-lateral aspect of the common carotid artery, through the bifurcation and should be extended into the internal carotid artery as far as the termination of the disease. Usually the first 1–2 cm of the internal carotid is opened but more extensive prolongation is sometimes required. Blind extraction of the distal limits of the plaque should not be performed and the final junction between the endarterectomised segment and normal intima should be fashioned under direct vision. In the majority of cases the disease peters out to give a smooth transition distally and only rarely does the intima require pinning with sutures at this point.

The external carotid artery may also be associated with the stenotic process and it should be carefully endarterectomised routinely during internal carotid endarterectomy. Occasionally, in the presence of an occluded internal carotid artery, local external carotid rebore may benefit collateral circulation (Conolly and Stemmer 1973). The arteriotomy is closed with direct continuous suture and significant narrowing rarely occurs (Angell-James and Lumley 1974). Occasionally technical considerations contra-indicate direct closure and a vein patch graft may then be used. Before the arteriotomy is finally closed all vessels are back bled and the lumen allowed to fill to exclude air bubbles. The declamping sequence is important and the external carotid and common carotid clamps are removed first. This allows the endarterectomised segment to be well flushed into the external carotid circuit and minimises the risk of minor residual debris taking the internal carotid route.

Per-operative arteriography at the completion of the procedure has been advocated by Smith (1974) and Rosental *et al.* (1973). The technique is, however, time consuming and not always practicable. Keitzer *et al.* (1972) prefer monitoring with a Doppler scan at the time of operation and we routinely use an electromagnetic flowmeter to confirm that the endarterectomy has achieved satisfactory haemodynamic results (Terry and Taylor 1974).

Provided a technically satisfactory endarterectomy is done recurrent stenosis is exceptionally rare (Blaisdell *et al.* 1967). Javid *et al.* (1974) reported only seven cases of re-stenosis in their extensive experience and these were thought to be due to incompleted removal of the distal segment of atheromatous plaque at the first operation. We have only encountered one case of re-stenosis and that was of non-atheromatous origin and occurred in a female of 31 years with a mucinoid degeneration of the artery.

The patient should be carefully monitored in the immediate post-operative period, with particular regard to the blood pressure which may be abnormally labile for the first 24 hours. This is probably due to interference with sinus nerve activity either directly or by the removal of the stent-like atheromatous core accross the carotid bifurcation (Wade *et al.* 1970, Angell-James and Lumley 1974). The latter authors showed that the operation of carotid endarterectomy changed the mechanical properties of the arterial wall, there being an overall increase in diameter and a reduction in distensability. These changes were in turn reflected in the recorded change of spontaneous sinus nerve activity and the systemic blood pressure. They suggested that the sinus nerve and carotid baroreceptor region should be carefully preserved during carotid endarterectomy

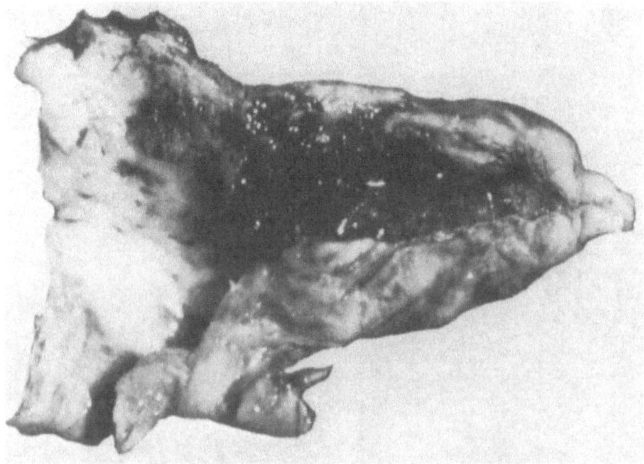

Fig. 5. Carotid endarterectomy specimen, note the extensive thrombus within the lumen

to prevent reflex post-operative hypertension. Reflex induced hypotension is most easily controlled by transfusion of whole blood and bradycardia by the administration of atropine. Post-operative hypertension is usually best treated conservatively or by sedation.

In patients with bilateral stenosis the symptomatic side is operated upon first. Synchronous carotid endarterectomy should not be performed and an interval of two weeks between sides is advisable.

Aneurysms of the Extra-Cranial Carotid Artery

Aneurysms of the extra-cranial carotid system are rare and Beall *et al.* (1962) found only seven such cases in 2,300 operations performed for aneurysm in their institution. Atherosclerosis and trauma are the most frequent causative factors, but occasional cases of mycotic aneurysm (Ledgerwood and Lucas 1974) cystic medial necrosis (Barnes and Jacoby 1962) and Marfan's syndrome (Hardin 1962) have been reported. The common carotid artery is involved twice as frequently as the internal or external carotid artery (Coleman and Kittle 1973). The usual presentation is of a symptomless pulsatile cervical mass. In this context mention should be made of the "spurious aneurysm" which presents as a pulsating swelling above the right sterno-clavicular joint in elderly hypertensive women.

This common entity is not a true aneurysm and is due to elongation and tortuosity of the innominate artery. It requires no treatment apart from control of the hypertension. True aneurysms may cause symptoms by rapid expansion or rupture. Rittenhouse *et al.* (1972) described a patient in whom a carotid aneurysm caused airway obstruction and eventual rupture into the oropharynx and we have had to undertake an emergency operation for a similar situation. Neurological symptoms may be the presenting feature secondary to cerebral embolisation by thrombus originating in the aneurysm sac (Weißman and Rankow 1968,

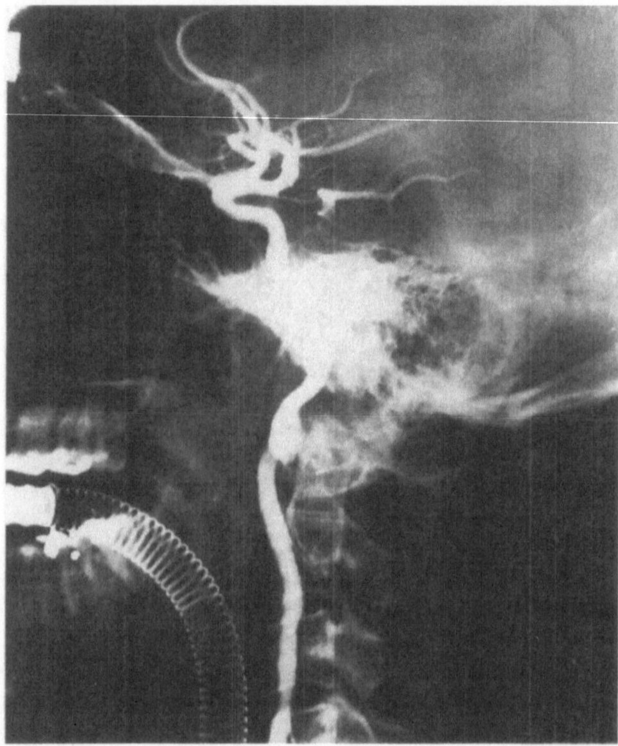

Fig. 6. Left carotid arteriogram of a 30 year old male patient showing an aneurysm of the internal carotid artery at the level of the atlas. The patient presented with a right sided hemiparesis and dysphasia. Four years previously he had been involved in a road traffic accident in which the left side of his neck had hit the steering wheel

Boddie 1972). Traumatic false aneurysm of the carotid system may follow either open or closedinjury (Deysine *et al.* 1969). They enlarge sl owly and the first indication of their presence may be TIA's. We have recently treated a young man who presented with a partial right sided stroke and who had suffered a severe closed contusion of the left side of the neck in a road accident four years previously. Angiography revealed a small aneurysm of the distal left internal carotid (Fig. 6). Carotid aneurysm, untreated, carries a bad prognosis and Winslow (1926) reported that 71% of 106 patients with untreated internal carotid aneurysm died of complications of the aneurysm.

Whenever possible resection of the aneurysm with restoration of continuity should be carried out (Rittenhouse *et al.* 1972). With common carotid aneurysms resection with end-to-end anastomosis is sometimes practicable (Kianouri 1967, Raphael *et al.* 1963), but usually an interposition graft will be required. Synthetic grafts may be used but autogenous vein is probably the best material for this purpose. The commonest complication of such surgery is a cerebro-vascular accident (Rittenhouse *et al.* 1972) and in order to minimise this risk the use of an intraluminal shunt is advised (Coleman and Kittle 1973).

Acute Carotid Injuries

Involvement of the carotid arteries in trauma to the cervical region presents certain difficulties in management and the problems have been well presented in a recent report by Thal *et al.* (1974). They discussed a series of 60 patients with carotid damage, the majority following penetrating injury, from gunshot or stab wounds. 65% of these injuries occurred on the left side and 80% involved the common carotid artery. Arterial laceration was the commonest injury with complete vessel transection in 18%, and the presence of an enlarging haematoma was the usual indication for operation. 19 (32%) of their 60 patients had developed a neurological deficit prior to operative treatment and this was severe in 13 (22%) patients. Restoration of arterial continuity was accomplished in the majority of patients with an overall mortality of 8.3%. The mortality was highest in patients with a severe pre-operative neurological deficit and it is likely that revascularisation of a fresh cerebral infarct was the responsible factor. These authors suggest that in patients with carotid injury and a severe neurological deficit angiographic assessment of carotid flow should be carried out. If flow is uninterrupted it is probably safe to repair the vessel. If, however, the distal segment is not patent, repair with restoration of flow carries too great a risk of cerebral oedema and arterial ligation should be undertaken.

Other operative procedures occasionally indicated on the carotid artery are the release of bands, the resection of the diseased areas with end-to-end anastomosis, or segmental replacement, and re-implanting or re-fashioning of the carotid bifurcation. More extensive exposure may be obtained by detaching the sterno-mastoid from the base of the skull by resecting the lower portion of the parotid gland, by dividing the stylo-hyoid or posterior belly of the digastric muscles and by dividing the angle of the mandible. Should neurological symptoms occur in a patient with fibro-muscular hyperplasia the most satisfactory form of operative treatment is carefully graded intraluminal dilatation (Morris *et al.* 1968).

Vertebral Arteries and Aortic Arch

Innominate endarterectomy was first undertaken by Davis *et al.* in 1956 and vertebral reconstruction by Crawford *et al.* (1958). Initially stenoses of the great vessels at the aortic arch were treated by bypass grafting (De Bakey *et al.* 1958, Crawford *et al.* 1962). A supra-clavicular approach, however, had been suggested by Lyons and Galbraith (1957) who introduced carotico-subclavian bypass procedures. In 1969 Crawford *et al.* compared the mortality of intra- and extra-thoracic corrective procedures for stenotic lesions of the aortic arch vessels and showed that the mortality of the extra-thoracic procedure was only 5.2% in contrast to a mortality of 22.2% in the direct approach. Harper *et al.* (1967) advised side-to-side anastomosis of the carotid and subclavian vessels. Theories that proximal bypass procedures may steal blood from the distribution of the feeding vessel were shown to be unfounded by Lord and Erenfeld (1969). These authors were able to show that flow was proportionally increased in the supplying vessel to a bypass and their work has subsequently been confirmed by Barner *et al.* (1971).

Intra-thoracic procedures are now usually limited to stenosis or occlusion of more than one of the main branches of the aortic arch. In these cases the graft can usually be taken off the aortic arch with a side-biting clamp for a bypass procedure, this being preferred to local endarterectomy when proximal control is usually necessary.

Moore *et al.* (1967) were able to disobliterate 7 of 10 common carotid artery occlusions retrogradely from arteriotomies made in the neck, while Javid *et al.* (1974) were successful in restoring flow in all of 7 similar patients. In aortic arch stenotic disease an alternative approach is to fashion uni or bilateral axillo-femoral bypasses (Sproul 1971).

Most extra-thoracic corrective procedures for aortic arch stenosis involve the insertion of short dacron or longer vein bypasses. These procedures usually require exposure of one or both subclavian arteries in the root of the neck. This is obtained through a transverse incision above the medial half of the clavicle dividing platysma, the lateral head of the sterno-mastoid muscle and the omohyoid muscle with its adjacent pad of fat. The phrenic nerve is retracted prior to division of the scalenus anterior muscle close to its attachment on the first rib. More extensive exposure can be obtained by totally dividing the lower end of the sterno-mastoid and resecting the proximal portion of the clavicle. Special care must be given during the exposure of the subclavian artery, to the brachial plexus, adjacent veins and the pleura. Heparinisation is again desirable before cross-clamping and shunting may be indicated. Occasionally the contralateral subclavian artery has to be used as the blood source for a diseased subclavian; a subclavian-to-subclavian bypass being undertaken (Finkelstein *et al.* 1972, Forestner *et al.* 1972). Alternatively a subcutaneous axillary-axillary bypass can be inserted (Mozersky *et al.* 1973). Bypass procedures may be combined with endarterectomy of one or both carotid bifurcations. Operators unfamiliar with this field should take particular care of the subclavian artery which is very thin and an easily damaged vessel. Carotico-axillary rather than carotico-subclavian bypass may be preferred for this reason.

Direct surgery on the vertebral artery is rarely indicated. Its contribution to total cerebral blood flow may be only one tenth of that of the carotid system and thus an isolated stenosis is unlikely to produce cerebral symptoms by a marked reduction in cerebral blood flow. When a stenosis is accompanied by a carotid lesion, relief of the carotid lesion is usually satisfactory in alleviating the patient's symptoms (Blaisdell *et al.* 1969). If the symptoms are due to embolism from a vertebral stenosis then the artery may be ligated, provided alternative channels are undiseased. Endarterectomy of the vertebral artery is usually limited to the proximal two centimetres, and the origin may be endarterectomised through a subclavian arteriotomy or alternatively a venous patch may be placed across it.

The techniques of extra-intracerebral revascularisation are considered elsewhere in this text.

Results

The results of surgery for strokes have markedly improved since the introduction of these procedures in the early 1950's. Safe anaesthetic and operative techniques have been established, although as already intimated these vary in different centres. Above all, clear indications now exist as to which group of patients should be selected for surgery and the relative value of surgery over conservative treatment has been assessed in a randomised series by the joint study of extra-cranial arterial occlusion (Fields *et al.* 1970). The overall mortality in patients with TIA's in the latter series was 3.5% with a 7.7% post-operative stroke rate. In this combined series, however, there was marked variation between institutions and the writers concluded that the operative mortality in specialised centres should be around, or less than, 1% and the morbidity less than 4% in this group of patients. De Weese *et al.* (1973) reported the five years results of 103 patients operated on for TIA's. At 30 days post-operatively 79% of the patients were asymptomatic, 15% had experienced an initial TIA and there were six patients with persistent neurological defects, two of them being severe whereas one patient had died. Studying the same group at five years post-operatively, 34 patients had died, a quarter due to myocardial infarction. The mortality was much higher in the over 60 age group of patients and in hypertensive and diabetic patients. Six of the eight patients with combined atherosclerotic heart disease and diabetes had died in the series. Five of the patients had died of strokes, one being a patient with an infected false aneurysm at the operation site which required proximal ligation. Two of the initial six patients with persistent post-operative neurological defects had died and one of the patients had died of stroke symptoms referable to the non-operated side. Of the 68 survivors, four patients had mild strokes, two moderate and one severe, and in the five year follow-up period, 17 patients had undergone contralateral carotid endarterectomy, 12 for TIA's and five for asymptomatic cervical bruits.

Thompson (1973 b) reported on the surgical results of 537 patients with TIA's. The operative mortality was 0.7% with a 1.5% incidence of permanent post-operative neurological defects. There was a 5% overall long term incidence of strokes, these including fatal and non-fatal episodes. This author considered that these figures showed a seven-fold reduction of severe strokes when compared with the expected natural history of the disease. Thompson (1973 b) emphasised that although the long term mortality rates in operative and non-operative stroke patients had not been extensively studied, except by the joint study (Fields *et al.* 1970), the reduced post-operative stroke rate in the operative group markedly affected the quality of life which the patients subsequently led.

De Weese *et al.* (1973) in their series of patients with TIA's further studied improvement of their patients in relation to the initial symptomatology. Of the 88 patients who they considered presented with classical TIA's, 76 were subsequently free of these symptoms, whereas only two of the 15 patients with atypical symptoms such as dizziness, syncopy, headache, seizures and confusion were relieved of their symptoms by the operative procedure. Fields *et al.* (1970) also commented on the failure of surgery to relieve non-classical symptoms. From these figures, therefore, one would conclude that surgery is the treatment of choice for patients with classical TIA's.

The work of Thompson and Patman (1970) and Javid *et al.* (1970) on the natural history of patients with asymptomatic bruits has already been referred to. Thompson (1973 a) compared conservative and surgical treatment of two groups of patients with asymptomatic bruits (the patients had not been randomly allocated). Of the 92 patients in the non-operative group over a 10 year period, 26% developed TIA's and 19% went on to persistent strokes. That is, 45% suffered subsequent neurological symptoms. Of the operative group of 66 patients undergoing 98 elective operations for asymptomatic bruits, there was no operative mortality, there were two operative strokes, one being severe, and in the late follow-up of these patients there were two late strokes, one being severe. There was no neurological mortality in the group. From these figures Thompson advised surgical treatment of asymptomatic carotid disease where there was bilateral or progressive disease, in unilateral severe stenosis, when the disease was related to the dominant hemisphere and when the patient was young. Possible contraindications are extensive cardiac or peripheral vascular disease, multiple lesions and increasing age. Follow-up on asymptomatic patients by Javid *et al.* (1971) showed no operative mortality, but a 3.6% morbidity. 90% of these patients, however, remained asymptomatic over a six to eight year follow-up.

The necessity to perform carotid endarterectomy prior to major surgery in a patient with asymptomatic disease is less well supported, although undertaken by a number of vascular units. Treiman *et al.* (1973) had no post-operative deaths from strokes in a group of 240 patients with asymptomatic cervical bruits undergoing surgery for abdominal aortic aneurysms. Bernhard *et al.* (1972) reported 16 patients who underwent combined endarterectomy and coronary artery bypass procedures, with no ensuing mortality and minimal morbidity.

Surgery in the acute developing phase of a stroke is now generally not undertaken or recommended. Blaisdell *et al.* (1969) reported a 42% mortality in a group of patients operated on within two weeks of an acute episode. Possible exceptions to this rule are a sudden occlusion occurring after angiography or when a large amount of free thrombus is radiologically demonstrated at the carotid bifurcation. Immediate post-operative occlusion of an endarterectomised vessel accompanied by progression of neurological symptoms has also been advocated as an indication for further surgery by some authors (Dye and Brown 1973). The chances of restoring patency of an occluded internal carotid vessel are increased with early operation, but so are the risks of haemorrhage into a recent infarct (Bruetman *et al.* 1963). Thompson *et al.* (1967) were able to restore flow in an occluded vessel in 40% of patients but the subsequent mortality in this situation was 6.2%.

Surgery offers little in the way of recovery to the patient with an established stroke, although some degree of mental improvement has been reported by most authors and quantitated by others (Perry *et al.* 1975). When reviewing surgery in patients with completed strokes, Dye and Brown (1973) reported that 35% patients improved, 20–30% of patients were unchanged, 10–20% were worse and the operative mortality was 15–30%. An operative mortality rate of 45% was recorded in the joint study (Blaisdell *et al.* 1969) in patients with an occluded carotid artery and associated residual neurological damage, when subsequent surgery was undertaken for TIA's related to the patent carotid vessel. Patterson (1974) however, found that in 23 similar patients there was no operative mortality and 17 of these patients were alive and 15 had no further symptoms 30 months later. Three patients had died and three had been lost to follow-up. Wylie and Ehrenfeld (1970) reported 70% relief of symptoms in patients with unilateral occlusion and TIA's related to the contralateral carotid stenosis. The variation in these results perhaps highlights the difference between the various schools.

Experience in non-atheromatous carotid artery disease is limited and critical assessment of the results is consequently difficult. The recommendations of Rundles and Kimbell (1969) in relation to kinks, however, is that these should only be operated on if the arterial lumen is reduced by more than 40% and in the absence of other possible causative lesions.

The reduced mortality of surgery for aortic arch conditions following the emphasis on an extra-thoracic approach, has already been mentioned. Long term results in the subclavian steal syndrome are generally excellent. Wylie and Ehrenfeld (1970) reported that vertebral artery surgery provided 70% relief of symptoms and an improvement in a further 21% of these patients on five year follow-up. Javid *et al.* (1974) reported the results obtained in 47 patients undergoing carotid-subclavian bypass procedures, 12 of the patients had simultaneous carotid endarterectomies. There was no hospital mortality in the group but later thrombosis was observed in four grafts, there were two wound infections and two false aneurysms. One of the patients developed a stroke from an associated carotid endarterectomy. The results of vertebral artery surgery from the same authors showed restoration of flow in 19 of 20 patients. There was temporary aggravation of symptoms in two patients, but no mortality and no severe neurological sequelae.

Conclusion

Experience accumulated on surgical treatment in patients with stroke syndromes since the initiation of these procedures in the early 1950's is such that distinct guidelines can now be laid down on the advisability of surgical treatment. Surgery should be the treatment of choice in patients with TIA's and a proven extra-cranial stenotic lesion, and in this group of patients the operative mortality should be in the order of 1% and severe neurological sequelae less than 4%. Surgery should generally be avoided in the developing stroke, whereas in the patient with a completed stroke it must be realised that improvement of established neurological damage is unlikely. The treatment of TIA's in the limbs contralateral to established neurological damage will depend largely on the experience and preferences of individual units. The treatment of asymptomatic stenosis remains controversial. They represent a potential stroke hazard but to justify surgical correction operative mortality should be below 1% and complications no more than 2%.

References

Abercrombie, J., 1828: Pathological and practical researches on diseases of brain and spinal cord. Edinburgh: Waugh and Innes.

Acheson, J., Hutchinson, E. C., 1971: The natural history of focal cerebral vascular disease. Quart. J. Med. *40*, 15—23.

Alajouanine, T., Lhermitte, F., Gautier, J. C., 1960: Transient cerebral ischaemia attacks in atherosclerosis. Neurology *10*, 906—914.

Alpers, B. J., Berry, R. G., Paddison, R. H., 1959: Anatomical studies of the circle of Willis in normal brain. Arch. Neurol. Psych. *81*, 409—418.

Angell-James, J. E., Lumley, J. S. P., 1974: The effects of carotid endarterectomy on the mechanical properties of the carotid sinus and carotid sinus nerve activity in atherosclerotic patients. Brit. J. Surg. *61*, 805—810.

Barner, H. B., Kaiser, G. C., Willman, V. L., 1971: Haemodynamics of carotid-subclavian bypass. Arch. Surg. *103*, 248—251.

Barnes, W. T., Jacoby, G. E., 1962: Aneurysm of the common carotid artery due to cystic medial necrosis treated by excision and graft. Ann. Surg. *155*, 82—85.

Beall, A. C., Crawford, E. S., Cooley, D. A., DeBakey, M. E., 1962: Extracranial aneurysms of the carotid artery. Report of seven cases. Postgrad. Med. *32*, 93—102.

Bernhard, V. M., Johnson, W. D., Peterson, J. J., 1972: Carotid artery stenosis. Association with surgery for coronary artery disease. Arch. Surg. *105*, 837—840.

Blaisdell, W. F., Clauss, R. H., Galbraith, J. G., Imparato, A. M., Wylie, E. J., 1969: Joint study of extracranial arterial occlusion. IV. A review of surgical considerations. J. Amer. Med. Assoc. *209*, 1889—1895.

— Glickman, M., Trunkey, D. D., 1974: Ulcerated atheroma of the carotid artery. Arch. Surg. *108*, 491—496.

— Lim, R., Hall, A. D., 1967: Technical results of carotid endarterectomy. Arteriographic assessment. Amer. J. Surg. *114*, 239—246.

Bloodwell, R. D., Hallman, G. L., Keats, A. S., Cooley, D. A., 1968: Carotid endarterectomy without a shunt. Arch. Surg. *96*, 644—652.

Boddie, H. G., 1972: Transient ischaemic attacks and stroke due to extracranial aneurysm of internal carotid artery. Brit. Med. J. *iii*, 802—803.

Boysen, G., 1971: Cerebral blood flow measurement as a safeguard during carotid endarterectomy. Stroke *2*, 1—10.

Brawley, B. W., Strandness, D. E., Kelly, W. A., 1967: The physiologic response to therapy in experimental cerebral ischaemia. Arch. Neurol. *17*, 180—187.

Brice, J. G., Dowsett, D. J., Lowe, R. D., 1964: Haemodynamic effects of carotid artery stenosis. Brit. Med. J. *ii*, 1363—1366.

Broadbent, W. H., 1875: Absence of pulsation in both radial arteries: the vessels being full of blood. Clin. Soc. Trans. *8*, 165—168.

Brockenbrough, E. C., 1970: Quoted by Keitzer *et al.* 1972.

Bruetman, M. E., Fields, W. S., Crawford, E. S., DeBakey, M. E., 1963: Cerebral haemorrhage in carotid artery surgery. Arch. Neurol. *9*, 458—467.

Caccamise, W. C., Whitman, J. F., 1952: Pulseless disease: Preliminary Case Report. Amer. Heart J. *44*, 629—633.

Carrea, R., Molins, M., Murphy, G., 1955: Surgical treatment of spontaneous thrombosis of the internal carotid artery in the neck. Carotid-carotideal anastomosis: Report of a case. Acta Neurol. Latinoamer. *1*, 71—78.

Chiari, H., 1905: Über das Verhalten des Teilungswinkels der carotis communis bei der Endarteritis chronica deformans. Verhandl. d. Deutsch. Path. Ges. *9*, 326—330.

Chung, W. B., 1974: Long-term results of carotid artery surgery for cerebrovascular insufficiency. Amer. J. Surg. *128*, 262—268.

Coleman, P. G., Kittle, C. F., 1973: Aneurysms of the common carotid artery. Surg. Clin. North Amer. *53*, 231—240.

Conolly, J. E., 1973: Discussion in Moore *et al.* 1973.

— Stemmer, E. A., 1973: Endarterectomy of the external carotid artery. Its importance in the surgical management of extracranial cerebrovascular occlusive disease. Arch. Surg. *106*, 799—802.

Contorni, L., 1960: Il circolo collaterale vertebro-vertebrale nella obliterazione dell'arteria subclavia alla sua origine. Minerva Chir. *15*, 268—271.

Cooley, D. A., Al-Naaman, Y. D., Carton, C. A., 1956: Surgical treatment of arteriosclerotic occlusion of common carotid artery. J. Neurosurg. *13*, 500—506.

Cooper, A., 1836: Account of the first successful operation, performed on the common carotid artery for aneurysm, in the year 1808, with the post mortem examination, in 1821. Guy's Hospital Report *1*, 53—58.

Crawford, E. S., DeBakey, M. E., Fields, W. S., 1958: Roentgenographic diagnosis and surgical treatment of basilar artery. J. Amer. Med. Assoc. *168*, 509—516.

— — Morris, G. C., Cooley, D. A., 1962: Thrombo-obliterative disease of the great vessels arising from the aortic arch. J. Thoracic. Cardiovasc. Surg. *43*, 38—53.

— — — Howell, J., 1969: Surgical treatment of occlusion of the innominate, common carotid and subclavian arteries: a ten year experience. Surgery *65*, 17—31.

David, T. E., Humphries, A. W., Young, J. R., Beven, E. G., 1973: A correlation of neck bruits and arteriosclerotic carotid arteries. Arch. Surg. *107*, 729—731.

Davis, J. B., Grove, W. J., Julian, O. C., 1956: Thrombic occlusion of branches of aortic arch. Martorell's syndrome: Report of case treated surgically. Ann. Surg. *144*, 124—126.

DeBakey, M. E., Morris, G. C., Jordan, G. L., Cooley, D. A., 1958: Segmental thrombo-obliterative disease of branches of the aortic arch. J. Amer. Med. Assoc. *166*, 998—1003.

Denny-Brown, D., 1951: Treatment of recurrent cerebrovascular symptoms and the question of "vasospasm". Med. Clin. North Amer. *35*, 1457—1474.

— Meyer, J. S., 1957: The cerebral collateral circulation. 2. Production of cerebral infarction by ischaemic anoxia and its reversibility in early stages. Neurol. *7*, 567—579.

De Weese, J. A., Rob, C. G., Satran, R., Marsh, D. O., Joynt, R. J., Summers, D., Nichols, C., 1973: Results of carotid endarterectomies for transient ischaemic attacks—five years later. Ann. Surg. *178*, 258—264.

Deysine, M., Adiga, R., Wilder, J. R., 1969: Traumatic false aneurysm of the cervical internal carotid artery. Surgery *66*, 1004—1007.

Dye, W. S., Brown, C. M., 1973: Surgical correction of carotid and vertebral artery stenosis. Surg. Clin. North Amer. *53*, 241—251.

Eastcott, H. H. G., Pickering, G. W., Rob, C. G., 1954: Reconstruction of internal carotid artery in a patient with intermittent attacks of hemiplegia. Lancet *ii*, 994—996.

Fields, W. S., Maslenikov, V., Meyer, J. S., Hass, W. K., Remington, R. D., 1970: Joint study of extracranial arterial occlusion. V. Progress report on prognosis following surgery of non surgical treatment for transient cerebral ischaemic attacks and cervical carotid artery lesions. J. Amer. Med. Assoc. *211*, 1993—2003.

Finkelstein, N. M., Byer, A., Rush, B. R., 1972: Subclavian—subclavian bypass for subclavian steal syndrome. Surgery *71*, 142—145.

Fisher, C. M., 1951: Occlusion of the internal carotid artery. Arch. Neurol. Psychiat. (Chicago) *65*, 346—377.

— 1954: Occlusion of the carotid arteries: further experience. Amer. Med. Assoc. Arch. Neurol. Psychiat. *72*, 187—204.

— 1959: Observations of the fundus oculi in transient monocular blindness. Neurology *9*, 333—347.

Forestner, J. E., Ghosh, S. K., Bergan, J. J., Conn, J., 1972: Subclavian—subclavian bypass for correction of the subclavian steal syndrome. Surgery *71*, 136—141.

Frøvig, A. G., 1946: Bilateral obliteration of the common carotid artery. Acta Psychiat. Neurol. Suppl. 39.

Gomensoro, J. B., Maslenikov, V., Azambuja, N., Fields, W. S., Lemak, N. A., 1973: Joint study of extracranial arterial occlusion. VIII. Clinical—radiographic correlation of carotid bifurcation lesions in 177 patients with transient cerebral ischaemic attacks. J. Amer. Med. Assoc. *224*, 985—991.

Gowers, W. R., 1875: On a case of simultaneous embolism of central retinal and middle cerebral arteries. Lancet *ii*, 794—796.

Hamby, W. B., 1952: Intracranial aneurysms. Springfield, Illinois: Thomas.

Hardin, C. A., 1962: Successful resection of carotid and abdominal aneurysms in two related patients with Marfan's syndrome. New England J. Med. *267*, 141—142.

Harper, J. A., Golding, A. L., Mazzei, E. A., Cannon, J. A., 1967: An experimental haemodynamic study of the subclavian steal syndrome. Surg. Gynec. Obst. *124*, 1212—1218.

Hayes, R. J., Levinson, S. A., Wylie, E. G., 1972: Intraoperative measurement of carotid back pressure as a guide to operative management for carotid endarterectomy. Surgery *72*, 953—960.

Hobson, R. W., Wright, C. B., Sublett, J. W., Fedde, C. W., Rich, N. M., 1974: Carotid artery back pressure and endarterectomy under regional anaesthesia. Arch. Surg. *109*, 682—687.

Houser, O. W., Baker, H. L., 1968: Fibromuscular dysplasia and other uncommon diseases of the cervical carotid artery: angiographic aspects. Amer. J. Roentgenol. *104*, 201—212.

Hunt, J. R., 1914: The role of the carotid arteries in the causation of vascular lesions of the brain, with remarks on certain special features of the symptomatology. Amer. J. Med. Sci. *147*, 704—713.

Javid, H., Dye, W. S., Hunter, J. A., Najafi, H., Goldin, M. D., Serry, C., 1974: Surgical treatment of cerebral ischaemia. Surg. Clin. North Amer. *54*, 239—255.

— Ostermiller, W. E., Hengesh, J. W., Dye, W. S., Hunter, J. A., Najafi, H., Julian, O. C., 1970: Natural history of carotid bifurcation atheroma. Surgery *67*, 80—86.

— — — — — — — 1971: Carotid endarterectomy for asymptomatic patients. Arch. Surg. *102*, 389—391.

Jennett, W. B., Harper, A. M., Gillespie, F. C., 1966: Measurement of regional cerebral blood flow during carotid ligation. Lancet *ii*, 1162—1163.

Karp, H. R., Heyman, A., Heyden, S., Bartel, A. G., Tyroler, H. A., Hames, C. G., 1973: Transient cerebral ischaemia: prevalence and prognosis in a biracial rural community. J. Amer. Med. Assoc. *225*, 125—128.

Kartchner, M. M., McRae, L. P., Morrison, F. D., 1973: Noninvasive detection and evaluation of carotid occlusive disease. Arch. Surg. *106*, 528—535.

Keitzer, W. F., Lichti, E. L., DeWeese, M. S., 1972: Clinical evaluation and correction of carotid artery occlusive disease. Use of the Doppler ultrasonic flowmeter. Amer. J. Surg. *124*, 697—700.

Kendell, R. E., Marshall, J., 1963: Role of hypotension in the genesis of transient focal cerebral ischaemic attacks. Brit. Med. J. *ii*, 344—348.

Kenyon, J. R., Thomas, A. B. W., Goodwin, D. P., 1972: Heparin protection for the brain during carotid artery surgery. Lancet *ii*, 153—154.

Kety, S. S., Schmidt, C. F., 1948: The effects of altered arterial tension of carbon dioxide and oxygen on cerebral blood flow and cerebral oxygen consumption of normal young men. J. Clin. Invest. *27*, 484—492.

Kianouri, M., 1967: Extracranial carotid aneurysm: Treatment by excision and end to end anastomosis. Ann. Surg. *165*, 152—156.

Kollarits, C. R., Lubow, M., Hissong, S. L., 1972: Retinal strokes. 1. Incidence of carotid atheroma. J. Amer. Med. Assoc. *222*, 1273—1275.

Lassen, N. A., Pálvölgyi, R., 1968: Cerebral steal during hypercapnia and inverse reaction during hypocapnia observed by the 133 xenon technique in man. Scand. J. Clin. Lab. Invest., Suppl. 102. XIII D.

Ledgerwood, A. M., Lucas, C. E., 1974: Mycotic aneurysm of the carotid artery. Arch. Surg. *109*, 496—498.

Leech, P. J., Miller, J. D., Fitch, W., Barker, J., 1974: Cerebral blood flow, internal carotid artery pressure and the EEG as a guide to the safety of carotid ligation. J. Neurol. Neurosurg. Psych. *37*, 854—862.

Lord, R. S. A., Ehrenfeld, W. K., 1969: Carotid-subclavian bypass: a haemodynamic study. Surgery *66*, 521—526.

Lyons, S. C., Galbraith, G., 1957: Surgical treatment of atherosclerotic occlusion of the internal carotid artery. Ann. Surg. *146*, 487—498.

Machleder, H. I., 1973: Evaluation of patients with cerebrovascular disease using the Doppler ophthalmic test. Angiology *24*, 374—381.

— Barker, W. F., 1972: Stroke on the wrong side. Use of the Doppler ophthalmic test in cerebral vascular screening. Arch. Surg. *105*, 943—947.

— — 1974: External carotid artery shunting during carotid endarterectomy. Arch. Surg. *108*, 785—788.

Marshall, J. M., 1969: In: "Extra-cranial cerebro-vascular disease and its management". Ed. Gillespie, J. A. London: Butterworth.

Martorell, F., Farbré, J., 1944: El sindrome de obliteracion de los troncos supra aorticos. Medicinia Clinica *2*, 26—30.

Millikan, C. H., Siekert, R. G., Shick, R. M., 1955: Studies in cerebrovascular disease. V. The use of anticoagulants drugs in the treatment of intermittent insufficiency of the internal carotid arterial system. Proc. Staff Meet. Mayo Clin. *30*, 578—586.

Moniz, E., Lima, A., DeLacerda, R., 1937: Hémiplégies par thrombose de la carotide interne. Presse Med. *45*, 977—980.

Moore, W. S., Blaisdell, F. W., Hall, A. D., 1967: Retrograde thrombectomy for chronic occlusion of the common carotid artery. Arch. Surg. *95*, 664—673.

— Hall, A. D., 1969: Carotid artery back pressure: a test of cerebral tolerance to temporary carotid occlusion. Arch. Surg. *99*, 702—710.

— Yee, J. M., Hall, A. D., 1973: Collateral cerebral blood pressure. An index of tolerance to temporary carotid occlusion. Arch. Surg. *106*, 520—523.

Morris, G. C., Lechter, A., De Bakey, M. E., 1968: Surgical treatment of fibromuscular disease of the carotid arteries. Arch. Surg. *96*, 636—643.

Mozersky, D. J., Sumner, D. S., Barnes, R. W., Strandness, D. E., 1973: Subclavian revascularization by means of a subcutaneous axillary—axillary graft. Arch. Surg. *106*, 20—23.

Paget, D. H., 1944: The circle of Willis, its embryology and anatomy. In: "Intracranial Arterial Aneurysms". Dandy, W. E. New York: Comstock.

Patterson, J. L., Heyman, A., Battey, L. L., Ferguson, R. W., 1955: Threshold of response of the cerebral vessels of man to increase blood carbon dioxide. J. Clin. Invest. *34*, 1857—1864.

Patterson, R. H., 1974: Risk of carotid surgery with occlusion of the contralateral carotid artery. Arch. Neurol. *30*, 188—189.

Perez-Borja, L., Meyer, J. S., 1965: Electrocephalographic monitoring during reconstructive surgery of the neck vessels. Electroencephalogr. Clin. Neurophysiol. *18*, 162—169.

Perry, P. M., Drinkwater, J. E., Taylor, G. W., 1975: Cerebral function before and after carotid endarterectomy. Brit. Med. J. *4*, 215—216.

Pickering, G. W., 1948: Transient cerebral palsy in hypertension and in cerebral embolism. J. Amer. Med. Assoc. *137*, 423—430.

Raphael, H. A., Bernatz, P. E., Spittell, J. A., Ellis, F. H., 1963: Cervical carotid aneurysms: Treatment by excision and restoration of arterial continuity. Amer. J. Surg. *105*, 771—778.

Reivich, M., 1961: A new vascular syndrome—"The subclavian steal". New Eng. J. Med. *265*, 912—913.

— Holling, H. E., Roberts, B., Toole, J. F., 1961: Reversal of blood flow through the vertebral artery and its effects on cerebral circulation. New Eng. J. Med. *265*, 878—885.

Rittenhouse, E. A., Radke, H. M., Sumner, D. E., 1972: Carotid artery aneurysm. Review of the literature and report of a case with rupture into the oropharynx. Arch. Surg. *105*, 786—789.

Rosental, J. J., Gaspar, M. R., Movius, H. J., 1973: Intraoperative arteriography in carotid thromboendarterectomy. Arch. Surg. *106*, 806—808.

Rundles, W. R., Kimbell, F. D., 1969: The kinked carotid syndrome. Angiography *20*, 177—194.

Russell, R. W. R., Cranston, W. I., 1961: Ophthalmodynamometry in carotid artery disease. J. Neurol. Neurosurg. Psychiat. *24*, 281—286.

Savory, W. S., 1856: Case of a young woman in whom the main arteries of both upper extremities and of the left side of the neck were throughout completely obliterated. Med. Chir. Trans. *39*, 205—219.

Shimizu, K., Sano, K., 1951: Pulseless disease. J. Neuropath. Clin. Neurol. *1*, 37—47.

Siekert, R. G., 1970: Quoted Austin *et al.* 1974.

Smith, L. L., 1974: In discussion Chung, 1974.

Sproul, G., 1971: Femoral—axillary bypass for cerebral vascular insufficiency. Arch. Surg. *103*, 746—747.

Strully, K. J., Hurwitt, E. S., Blankenberg, H. W., 1953: Thromboendarterectomy for thrombosis of the internal carotid artery in the neck. J. Neurosurg. *10*, 474—482.

Sutherland, G. R., Donaldson, A. A., 1972: Persistant hypoglossal artery complicated by internal carotid artery stenosis. Clin. Radiol. *23*, 222—224.

Svien, H. J., Hollenhorst, R. W., 1956: Pressure in retinal arteries after ligation or occlusion of the carotid artery. Proc. Staff Meet Mayo Clin. *31*, 684—692.

Takayasu, M., 1908: A case with peculiar changes of the central retinal vessels. Acta Soc. Ophthal. Jap. *12*, 554.

Terry, H. J., Taylor, G. W., 1974: Quantitation of flow in femoropopliteal grafts. Surg. Clin. North Amer. *54*, 85—94.

Thal, E. R., Snyder, W. H., Hays, R. J., Perry, M. O., 1974: Management of carotid artery injuries. Surgery *76*, 955—962.

Thomas, G. I., Spencer, M. P., Jones, T. W., Edmark, K. W., Stavney, L. S., 1974: Noninvasive carotid bifurcation mapping. Its relation to carotid surgery. Amer. J. Surg. *128*, 168—174.

Thompson, J. E., 1973 a: The development of carotid artery surgery. Arch. Surg. *107*, 643—648.

— 1973 b: In discussion DeWeese *et al.* 1973.

— Austin, D. J., Patman, R. D., 1967: Endarterectomy of the totally occluded carotid artery for stroke: results in 100 operations. Arch. Surg. *95*, 791—801.

— Patman, R. D., 1970: Endarterectomy for asymptomatic carotid bruits. Heart Bull. 19, 116—120.

Todd, R. B., 1844: Account of a case of a dissecting aneurysm of the aorta innominata and right carotid arteries giving rise to suppression of urine and white softening of the brain. Medico-Chirurgical Transactions (2nd series) *27*, 301—324.

Treiman, R. L., Foran, R. F., Shore, E. H., Levin, P. M., 1973: Carotid bruit: significance in patients undergoing an abdominal aortic operation. Arch. Surg. *106*, 803—805.

Trojaborg, W., Boysen, G., 1973: Relation between EEG, regional cerebral blood flow and internal carotid artery pressure during carotid endarterectomy. Electroencephalogr. Clin. Neurophysiol. *34*, 61—69.

Virchow, R., 1856: Cited by Hager, H., 1962: Die Diagnose der Karotisthrombose durch den Augenarzt. Klin. Nbl. Augenheilk. *141*, 801—840.

Wade, J. G., Larson, C. P., Hickey, R. F., Ehrenfeld, W. K., Severinghaus, J. W., 1970: Effect of carotid endarterectomy on carotid chemoreceptor and baroreceptor function in man. New Eng. J. Med. *282*, 823—829.

Weissman, B. A., Rankow, R. M., 1968: Traumatic aneurysm of the common carotid artery. Arch. Otolaryngol. *88*, 543—546.

Wells, B. A., Keats, A. S., Cooley, D. A., 1963: Increased tolerance to cerebral ischaemia produced by general anaesthesia during temporary carotid occlusion. Surgery *54*, 216—223.

White, C. W., Allarde, R. R., McDowell, H. A., 1967: Anaesthetic management for carotid artery surgery. J. Amer. Med. Assoc. *202*, 1023—1027.

Winslow, N., 1926: Extracranial aneurysms of the internal carotid artery: Historical analysis of the cases registered up until August 1st, 1925. Arch. Surg. *13*, 689—729.

Wright, R. L., Sweet, W. H., 1962: Treatment of intracranial aneurysms by carotid occlusion: correlation of late clinical follow-up with pressure recordings. Trans. Amer. Neurol. Assoc. *87*, 158—162.

Wylie, E. J., Ehrenfeld, W. K., 1970: Extracranial occlusive cerebrovascular disease. Diagnosis and management. Philadelphia: Saunders and Co.

Wylie, W., 1974: In discussion Hobson *et al.* 1974.

Young, J. R., Humphries, A. W., Beven, E. G., de Wolfe, V. G., 1969: Carotid endarterectomy without shunt. Experience using hyperbaric general anaesthesia. Arch. Surg. *99*, 293—297.

Intrathecal Injection of a Neurolytic Solution for the Relief of Intractable Pain

J. RÉTIF

Department of Neurosurgery, University of Brussels (Belgium)

With 12 Figures

Contents

I. Introduction

The concept according to which the different nerve fibers (myelinated and unmyelinated fibers of various diameters) can be affected differently by various blocking or destructive agents has been the rationale for many attempts to relieve pain or spasticity.

Among these various agents we shall quote cold, heat, hypertonic saline, procaïne, alcohol and phenol. For example it has been shown that conduction velocity decreases more rapidly with cold in group A fibers than in group C fibers (de Jesus *et al.* 1973). These various agents, which are able either to selectively destroy certain groups of fibers, to inhibit function, or to reduce the conduction velocity in some fibers, were applied to different sites of the peripheral nervous system *e.g.* injection of alcohol to motor sites of the muscles, application of the agent to peripheral nerves or to nerve roots.

I. Cooper (1965) has tried a technique of isolated perfusion of a limb with

0.2% phenol solution in order to produce a specific neurotoxic effect upon various elements of the peripheral nervous system, mainly upon the small fibers of the gamma motor type.

Because of these different responses of the nervous fibers to various blocking agents (Gasser and Erlanger 1929), several therapeutic attempts have been performed but many of them were not repeated. However, the subarachnoid injection of chemical neurotoxic agents has gained a large usage which allows a valuable analysis of the method of chemical radicotomy.

II. Subarachnoid Injection of Alcohol

Neurotoxic substances placed in direct contact with nerve roots to interrupt fibers carrying pain, were first used in 1914 when Härtel described a method of intracranial injection of alcohol for treatment of idiopathic neuralgia of the trigeminal nerve. However, the now classic study of Dogliotti in 1931 is used as the standard reference for aspects concerning the subarachnoid injection of absolute alcohol. In his paper he described the use of a method that he devised in 1922 and reported curing cases of sciatica by injection of alcohol into the sacral cul-de-sac where it was in direct contact with the posterior roots.

This technique was used for a long time after it was reported by Dogliotti and enjoyed a certain degree of popularity (Stern 1934 and 1936; Salzstein 1934; Greenhill and Schmitz 1935; Abbott 1936; Poppen 1936; Russell 1936; Adson, 1937; Ottley 1938; Groff 1939; Todd 1939; Pitts and Browder 1939; Truelsen 1943; Ansbro 1950; Bonica 1954).

The principle, as described by Dogliotti, is based upon the fact that the painful stimulus can no longer reach the stimulation threshold of the central nervous pathways for pain if the number of nociceptive impulses is sufficiently reduced. He sought to destroy a certain number of the nervous fibers of the posterior spinal roots with alcohol.

1. Technique

Absolute alcohol which is lighter than cerebro-spinal fluid (having a specific gravity of 0.775 as compared to 1.006 for CSF), when injected by lumbar puncture or by sub-arachnoid puncture into a level other than the lumbar region, rises and floats at the highest spot in the sub-arachnoid space. Thus, whenever an injection is performed, the patient must be positioned in such a way that the painful region and the posterior spinal roots involved are as high as possible (Fig. 1 and 2), the needle, if at all possible, placed at the apex of the curve of the spinal column.

If the patient is lying on the healthy, non-painful side, the alcohol flows more directly and more efficiently towards the posterior roots if he bends 45° ventrally. It is always necessary to be certain that the head and hips are kept at a level lower than that of the injection. In this way the alcohol rises along the posterior roots into the arachnoid cul-de-sac. The patient should be kept in this position for at least 30 to 40 minutes after the injection before he is allowed to return to his bed.

Some 20 years ago we used Dogliotti's method, without any modification, using a fine or average diameter lumbar puncture needle (22 or 20 gauge, with a short bevel) in light of the fluid characteristics of alcohol. At the same time we attempted to inject the alcohol by the shortest possible route, performing the injection as close as possible to the posterior spinal roots corresponding to the painful dermatomes implicated in the pain syndrome (Brihaye, Rétif and Grégoire, 1961; Brihaye, Rétif and Grégoire, 1962) because alcohol is very easily diluted in CSF, diffusing very rapidly and extensively in the sub-arachnoid space.

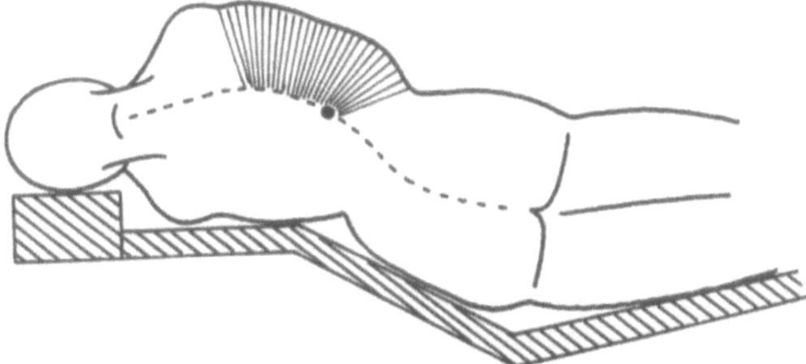

Fig. 1. Injection of alcohol at the level of the inferior third of the thorax (Th. 7, 8 and 9) for relief of thoracic pain projected in the middle third

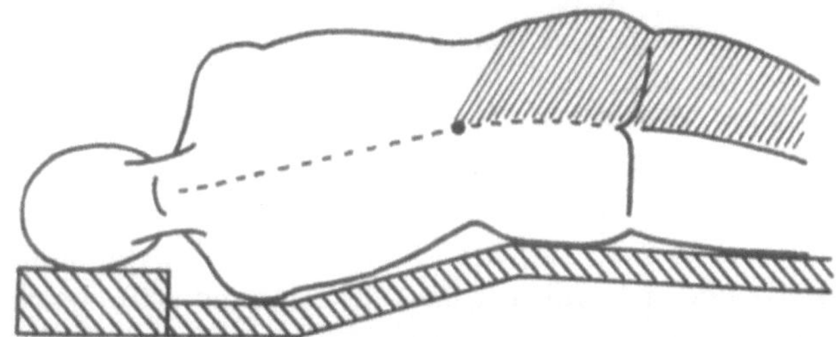

Fig. 2. Lumbar puncture for injection of alcohol at L 4—L 5 or L 5—S 1 level for relief of lumbo-sacral and sacral pain

Dogliotti's method was modified by some authors without, in our opinion, any particular advantage. The following modifications have been tried; Sloane (1935) mixed alcohol and CSF in the syringe before injection; Poppen (1936) performed two or three punctures at different vertebral levels; Ansbro (1950) placed, under radiographic control, a catheter in the sub-arachnoid space under consideration.

Tank, Dohn, and Gardner in 1963, and Derrick in 1970 described a prone position which made it possible to perform a bilateral lumbo-sacral alcoholisation at the same time: the patient lay on his stomach and the sacral cul-de-sac was punctured at the L 5—S 1 level. With the sacrum raised, 0.5 to 0.7 ml of alcohol was injected; the table was then tilted and the patient was then in a position where his head was at a lower level than the rest of the body.

2. *Results*

Our results can be summarized as follows:

Twenty four injections were performed on 15 patients (13 cancer patients, one painful spastic paraplegic, one case of post-zoster thoracic pain). We obtained

7 good results (4 almost complete disappearance of pain and 3 very satisfactory decrease in pain) and 8 failures.

We were not able to establish any correlation between the quality of the results and the radicular level at which the injection was performed (4 times at C 7—Th 1, 3 times at a high thoracic level, 9 times at a low thoracic level, 8 lumbar and lumbo-sacral). On the other hand, it was apparent that the quality of the results chiefly depended upon the quantity of alcohol injected. Thus, our 8 failures occurred when the quantity of fluid injected did not exceed 1 ml while the best results were obtained when the dose was between 2 to 3 ml.

We had complications in 4 out of 7 patients, each of whom received more than 1 ml of absolute alcohol, in the satisfactory results group.

Our series is very small, but the large number of failures (8 out of 15 patients: 55%) is noteworthy.

Some authors have been very satisfied with Dogliotti's method and have reported success rates ranging from 75 to 100% (Saltzstein, 1934; Stern, 1934; Greenhill and Schmitz, 1935; Abbott, 1936; Todd, 1939; Truelsen, 1943; Dogliotti, 1943, 1957). Derrick in 1970, reported 85% good results out of 322 patients, and only two permanent complications.

Other authors have reported results similar to ours or approximately 50 to 75% improvement (Russell, 1936; Peyton, Semansky, and Baker, 1937; Grant, 1941; Ansbro, 1950). In 106 patients suffering from intractable cancer pain, Hay, Yonezawa, and Derrick (1959) obtained total remission in 50% of their cases, partial remission in 33% and observed complications in only three cases.

Such varying results have also been found in more recent publications. For instance, Tank, Dohn, and Gardner in 1963 reported 53% good results, and 30% failures, the rest of their group being classified satisfactory. Kuzucu, Derrick, and Wilber (1966) reported that out of 322 patients with advanced cancer they had 58% with significant relief from pain, 26% with partial relief and 16% failure. These authors had better results at the upper thoracic or cervical level as compared to the lumbo-sacral level in spite of the technical difficulties of the procedure at a high level.

It is difficult to blame the technique, which is simple and easy to perform for the notable differences in results obtained by different authors. The quantity of alcohol injected certainly plays a role, as does the subjective nature of the perception of the therapeutic results.

We have never observed a delayed effect of alcohol, the action of which could be progressive, reaching a maximum sometimes even 24 hours after the injection (Dogliotti, 1943; Stern, 1934; Kuzucu *et al.*, 1966). At the moment of injection all our patients had an impression of heat, sometimes intense, in the corresponding territory, followed in a few minutes by analgesia to pin prick while pain sensation disappeared at the same time. Unfortunately, this effect was often only transitory, since the zone of analgesia shrinks within days, if not hours, after the injection, while at the same time the pain progressively reappears.

This fleeting "local anesthetic" effect, which can be seen with other neurotoxic substances injected into the sub-arachnoid space, probably depends upon the concentration of alcohol in cerebro-spinal fluid where its contacts the nerve roots. Alcohol, which is very soluble in CSF, is probably diluted rapidly and then does not sufficiently affect the roots in question.

The length of time during which there is relief of pain is variable. Some patients are free of pain for from 6 to 10 months, the average being 3 to 4 months. In many cases, however, this relief lasts only a few weeks at most.

There is no specific relationship between this effect and the diameter of the nerve fibers. It is not at all certain that the large fibers, which are more myelinated, are more slowly and less affected than the fine fibers as Olmsted and Hodgson in 1931 described it in peripheral nerves and Hariga *et al.* in 1966 in the medial popliteal nerve in cats. Alcohol, which has a demyelinizing and degenerating action on the axis cylinders of the posterior roots, does not have particular specificity for any fibers. Its maximum action extends from the periphery to the center of the nerve and appears to be simply proportional to its concentration (Hay *et al.* 1959).

3. Complications

The dilution of alcohol in the cerebro-spinal fluid is a fact but its role is much less negligible than the defenders of alcoholization would like to admit. This diffusion is less dangerous if no more than 1 ml is injected or if the amount is divided over several medullary levels by multiple punctures (Poppen, 1939; Derrick, 1970).

If a larger quantity of alcohol is injected, its action on the posterior roots, and as a result its effect on pain, will be greater but the amount of diffusion can be such that the risk of complications would no longer be negligible. Medullary complications, sometimes serious, have been reported (Russell, 1936; Peyton *et al.*, 1937; Todd, 1939; Groff, 1941; Truelsen, 1943; Hay *et al.*, 1959; Brihaye *et al.*, 1962) as well as complications, which are not infrequent, involving the anterior roots at the lumbar level, or spincter disorders (Hay *et al.*, 1959; Brihaye *et al.*, 1962).

Our complications consisted of 2 cases of peripheral type paresis of the lower limb, one of which was transitory in nature, one case of urinary retention which lasted until the patient died 5 months later, and one case of Brown-Séquard syndrome which was secondary to alcoholization for a Pancoast syndrome.

It is difficult to quantify the percentage of complications, but the risk of neurological sequelae is real and most authors who still use this technique reserve it for cancer patients in a poor general state already suffering from sphincter problems or with a short expectation of life.

The indications for the use of alcoholization for "benign" pains have almost completely disappeared because it is bound to end in failure after a certain length of time (intractable sciatica, post-zoster neuralgia, pain of osteo-arthritis of the hip).

In conclusion, sub-arachnoid injection of alcohol is a simple, rapid and relatively painless procedure which makes chemical posterior rhizotomy easy. The risk of complications is small provided that no more than 1 ml of solution is injected. The average duration of effectiveness is unfortunately variable, with success in only 50% of the cases unless a larger amount of absolute alcohol is used (2 ml or more). The length of pain sedation can be as much as 6 to 10 months or can last for only a few weeks. The mean length of time is 3 to 4 months. When a larger quantity of alcohol is used, the percentage of radiculo-medullary and sphincter problems increase prohibitively, which has led to a progressive decrease in the indications for the treatment for pain in cancer patients unless they have a short life expectancy or previous sphincter disturbances.

III. Subarachnoid Injection of Phenol

The technique of intra-thecal injection of alcohol which was practically no longer used except by anesthetists (Bonica, 1953; Derrick *et al.* 1959) would probably have disappeared if Maher, in 1955, had not revived an interest in it. He modified the principle by using a neurotoxic and neurolytic substance which was this time hyperbaric when compared to CSF and which diffused less slowly than alcohol in CSF. In searching for a substance which would produce a permanent anesthesia, he widely experimented with phenol in a viscous solution (Maher 1955, Brown 1958, Nathan 1959), later in myodil which was used for myelography, and finally in a glycerin solution (Mark *et al.* 1963).

1. Technique

The choice of the neurolytic substance remains phenol. Chlorocresol in a 2% solution in glycerin was also used by Maher (1963) but was not continued.

Fresh solutions of phenol in glycerin are generally recommended because the phenol degrades and loses its activity over a period of time. At that point the solution has a rose color. The pharmaceutical preparation of the solution should be from sterilized anhydrous glycerin and perfectly dehydrated phenol (Brown 1961) which must be freshly diluted in its solvent. The usual concentrations are from 5 to 7.5% in glycerin (the 5% solution is most often used) and from 5 to 10% in solution in liposoluble radio-opaque iodinated substances (Maher 1957, Nathan and Scott 1958, Mark *et al.* 1963). These latter preparations are now hardly ever used (Lourie and Vanasupa 1963, White 1965, White and Sweet 1969).

At one time solutions of phenol in glycerin containing, in addition, silver nitrate were used; this significantly increased the activity of the solution, but also its toxic nature, so much so that it was necessary to add water to the solution. This served only to ease and accelerate the diffusion of phenol in CSF (Maher 1957, 1960). Serious medullary accidents rapidly led to discontinuing the use of the mixture of drugs. It is known that the toxic effect on living tissues, and on nerves in particular, is variable according to the solvent used (Maher 1955, Brown 1958, Baxter and Schacherl 1962, Smith 1964, Knott, Katz, and Rubinstein 1969). Diffusion from an oily solution into cerebro-spinal fluid is slow; it is much more rapid from an aqueous solution, but the effects of this diffusion are poorly controlable, even for weak concentrations. The various substances which have been used have not shown any notable advantage over phenol which remains the most used product, glycerin remaining the solvent of choice.

The average quantity injected is 1 ml. This can be increased to 1.5 ml or even 2 ml at one time when it is injected far from the lumbo-sacral or brachial plexus. 2 ml seems to be the maximum quantity that can be injected at one time.

This technique of phenol solution in glycerin has been reviewed on numerous occasions by several different authors, but its general principles have not been substantially modified since Maher (Brown 1958, Mark *et al.* 1962, Stovner *et al.* 1972, Papo *et al.* 1968). It is this technique that was used for our patients.

The use of hyperbaric substances as the vehicle for the neurotoxic drug implies, in contrast to the technique of alcoholization, that the painful side be in the lower position. If the patient is in a lateral decubitus position, the vertebral column is laterally bent so that the nerve roots corresponding to the painful zone are in the lowest position and the injected material collects there by gravity.

The sub-arachnoid space is punctured at this lowest vertebral level with a needle which is sufficiently large (18 gauge) to enable injection of the high viscosity fluid.

Since the puncture is not always possible at the same level as that of the nerve roots involved, it can be performed either a few spaces higher or lower. In this case the patient is placed on a tilting table, inclined in a more or less cranial or caudal direction according to the individual case so that the phenol-glycerin solution can flow towards the nerve roots in question, situated at the lowest vertebral point (Figs. 3 to 8).

The head and the region of the cauda equina must be raised so that the phenol does not reach them by accident.

The lumbar puncture needles must be placed in a strictly median sagittal plane (Fig. 9) and at the moment of injection, the patient, who remains in a lateral decubitus position, should turn 35 to 45° backwards so that the phenol solution touches the posterior nerve roots as selectively as possible (Fig. 10).

In the case of ano-rectal pain the patient is placed in a sitting position and the puncture is performed at the L 5—S 1 level; the phenol is injected while the patient leans backwards approximately 40°.

The total quantity of material injected is approximately 1.0 to 1.5 ml, the injection being performed in a graduated fashion, in increments of approximately 0.4 ml. If necessary, the position of the patient and the tilting of the table can be modified in the light of the cutaneous hypoesthesia or even anesthesia which occurs within 30 to 40 seconds following the injection. On the average, 1 ml is injected at the lumbar and lumbo-sacral level, 2 ml can be injected into the sacral cul-de-sac in cases of anorectal pain and when sphincter problems are already present. Approximately 1.5 ml can also be injected at the thoracic and cervical levels.

A 5% solution is usually used, but a solution of 7.5% phenol in glycerin can be used if placed far from the plexuses, especially at thoracic and abdominal levels. Mark *et al.* (1962) went so far as to inject 7 to 8 ml of 10% solution in pantopaque.

The fractionated injection lasts for 20 to 30 minutes in general, the needle remaining in place during that time. After the injection the patient normally remains in the same position for 30 or 45 minutes, after which he can return to his bed, staying in the initial lateral position for at least 4 hours with his head supported by pillows.

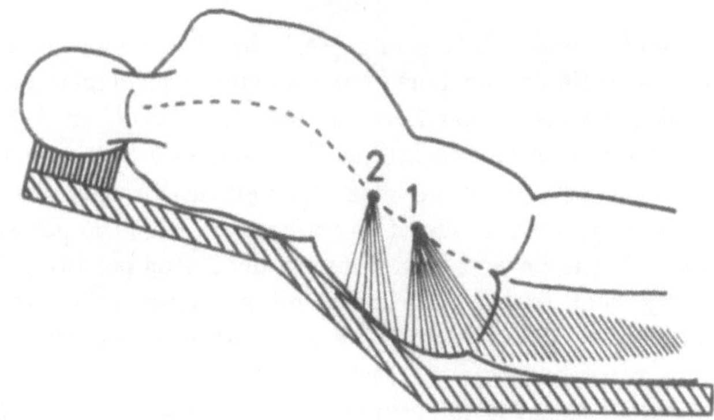

Fig. 3. *1* Lumbar puncture at L 5—S 1 level for unilateral sacral pain, *2* high lumbar puncture (L 1, L 2 or L 2—L 3) for lumbar pain. (Phenolization)

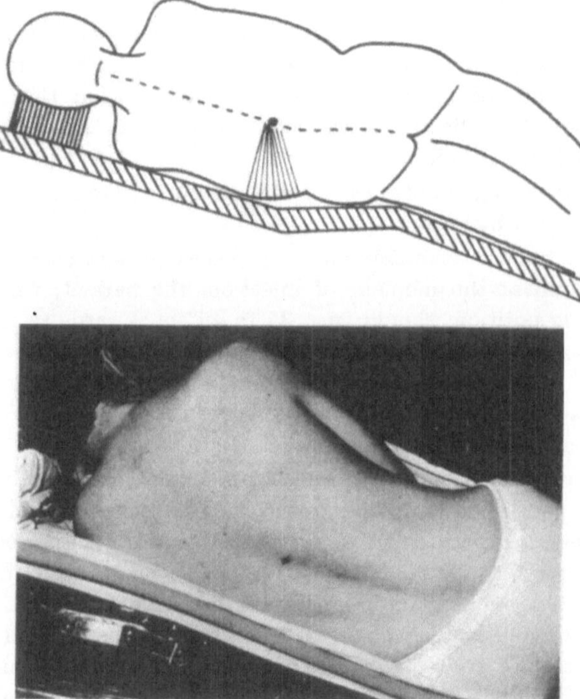

Fig. 4. Injection of phenol solution at a high lumbar or at a thoraco-lumbar level for relief of lumbar pain. The seat is raised for avoiding sacral roots

2. Rationale of the Method

Maher, using phenol for intra-thecal injections, was looking for an agent that would produce permanent anesthesia and based his whole theory on selective destruction by the neurolytic agent of the fine afferent fibers which are only slightly myelinated or non-myelinated, and on the fact that the large radicular fibers, which are highly myelinated, would be selectively spared from its action. Thus, only the fine C fibers which conduct pain would be selectively blocked in a

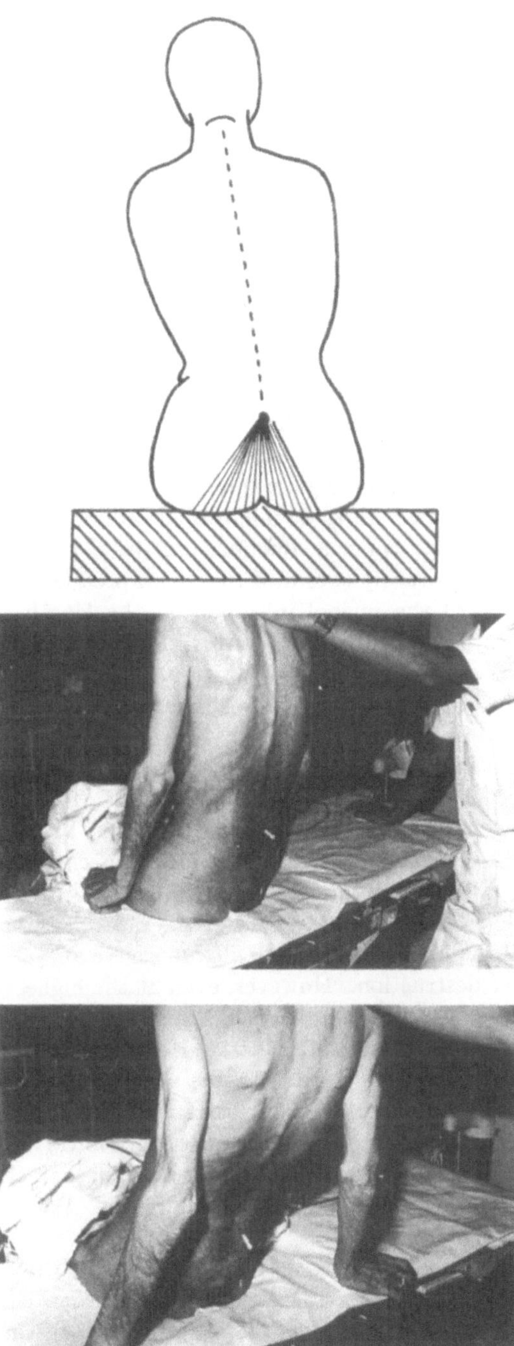

Fig. 5. Injection of phenol solution at L 5—S 1, patient in a sitting position, and afterwards leaning backwards 45° for relief of perianal and sacral pain

persistant fashion after the transitory local anesthetic effect had disappeared. The clinical result could correspond to the disappearance of pain without any, or hardly any, objective effect on sensation or mobility.

By an electrophysiologic study in cats Nathan and Sears (1960) were able to find that C fibers (pain) were the first to be blocked in a persistant manner, while conduction by A fibers was conserved or altered in only a temporary fashion. Iggo and Walsh (1960) were also able to show by electrophysiological methods that the fine radicular fibers were selectively blocked.

It was from clinical observations that such a selective destruction of the fine fibers by neurotoxic substances, and by phenol in particular, had been envisioned (Maher 1955 and 1957, Brown 1958 and 1961, Nathan and Scott 1958); in effect, these authors frequently found that the disappearance of pain was not necessarily accompanied by an objective decrease in touch or even pain sensitivity.

According to our experience, in the beginning, the phenol solution affects a large number of nerve fibers of different sizes coming from several different roots. This produces the rapidly induced (less than one minute) local anesthetic effect. After a relatively short time (15 to 60 minutes according to our experience) most of the nerve fibers recover their conduction, certain of them completely, others only partially, according to the extent of the lesion produced which is a function of the concentration of the phenol injected and the length of time the nerve fibers are in contact with the toxin. The relative number of damaged fibers will determine the extend of the objective analgesia and the anodyne effect. It is certain that a relatively large number of fibers must be destroyed before objective clinical sensory loss appears.

The selective destruction of fine fibers by phenol solution has, unfortunately, never been proven histologically (Steward and Lourie 1963). It is possible that the finest fibers are blocked before the larger ones, but fibers of all sizes are affected in a global fashion, as a function of the local concentration of phenol where it touches the nerve roots. All the histological studies performed have confirmed this notion of a global and variable injury of the radicular fibers. Generally the more concentrated the phenol solution, the more severe and extensive will be the lesion and radicular destruction. However, even at the highest concentrations, a large number of fibers of all sizes can remain intact, as we observed in one of our cases where we performed surgical posterior rhizotomy after phenol injection.

Relatively few papers have dealt with the study of the lesions produced by the intra-thecal injection of phenol in humans (Mark *et al.* 1962, Berry and Olszewski 1963, André-Balisaux and Gonsette 1963, Smith 1964, Hansebout and Cosgrove 1966) or even in animals (Baxter and Schacherl 1962, Stewart and Lourie 1963, Smith 1964, Papo *et al.* 1967, Knott *et al.* 1969, Schaumburg *et al.* 1970).

A histological study of nerve roots placed in contact with a phenol solution shows segmentary demyelinization, followed by Wallerian degeneration, which appears to be in direct relationship to the concentration of the solution and the length of the time. The root is in contact with this antiseptic and sclerosing substance; spinal roots are mainly affected; phenol does not appear to reach the spinal ganglia (Baxter and Schacherl 1962, Smith 1964).

The demyelinization appears in plaques, predominantly at the periphery,

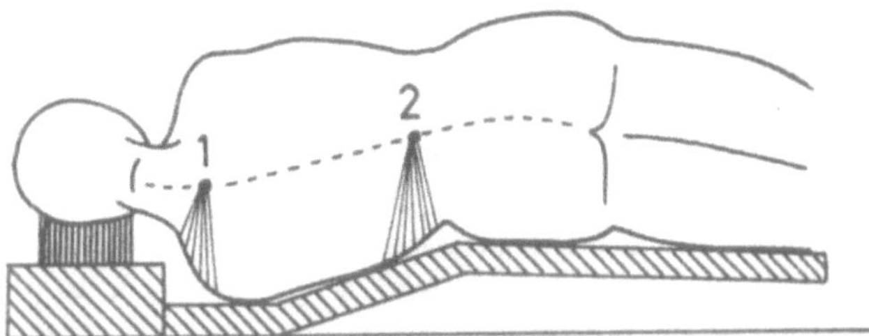

Fig. 6. *1* Injection of phenol solution at C 7—Th 1 or C 6—C 7 for pain of the left upper limb, *2* dorso-lumbar injection for low thoracic pain or thoraco-lumbar pain

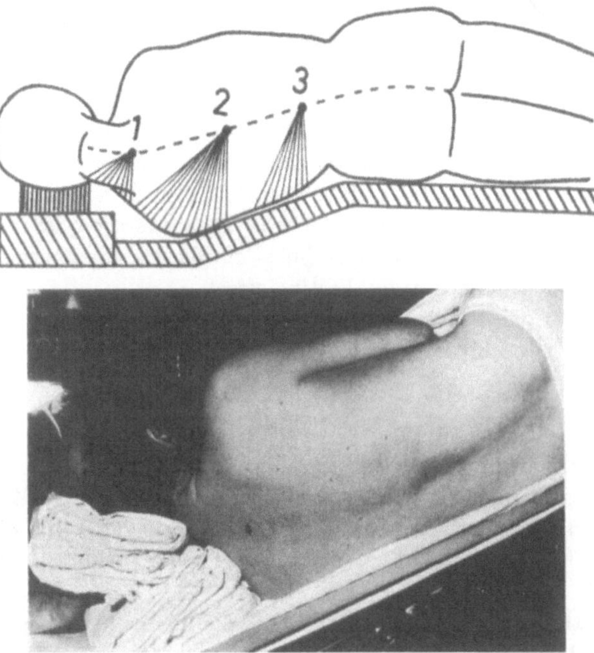

Fig. 7. *1* Injection of phenol-solution at C 5—C 6 or C 6—C 7 for low cervical pain, *2* injection at the middle thoracic level for high thoracic pain, *3* injection at the inferior thoracic level for pain in the middle third of the thorax

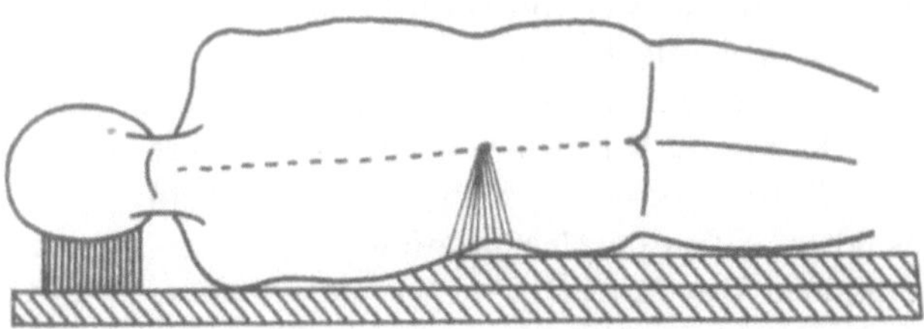

Fig. 8. High lumbar injection for thoraco-lumbar pain

and the axonal degeneration has the same distribution. The degeneration of fine fibers is the same as that of large ones (Fig. 11 and 12). According to Schaumburg *et al.* 1970, the large myelinated fibers are even more sensitive to the neurotoxic substances. This notion is in line with the frequent observation in our series of the existence of a global sensory deficit in the area corresponding to the suppression of pain. For us, the persistance of such a deficit is almost the guarantee of persistent pain relief, though this is contrary to the opinion of several authors (Maher 1955, Mark *et al.* 1963).

Thus, pathological study has not made it possible to verify the hypothesis of a selective lesion of the C fibers by intra-thecal injection of phenol. The radicular lesion predominates at the periphery, where the concentration of phenol is the greatest, and involves large fibers just as much as fine fibers.

Nathan, Sears, and Smith (1965) summarize the electrophysiological and histological data, trying to integrate it with clinical observations. Phenol, which is able to penetrate into tissues and coagulate protein, apparently has two actions. The first is a local anesthetic type of action which produces a temporary differential block; the second is related to a global, non-differenciated destruction. The durable clinical result on pain is the consequence of the quantitative suppression of function of a certain number of fibers of all sizes, myelinated or otherwise, rather than the consequence of qualitative effect.

These observations at least explain those cases in which early recurrence of pain contrasts with an initial, but fleeting, cutaneous analgesia.

3. Clinical Results

Numerous studies have followed those of Maher (1955, 1957, 1963, 1966) and the number of cases reported is quite large: almost 500 cases by Maher, 181 cases by Brown in 1961, 289 by Ciocatto 1967 (cited by Papo and Visca 1973); 180 cases by Papo and Visca in 1968, 352 cases by these same authors in 1973, 351 cases by Stovner and Endresen in 1972, etc.

Ever since the first cases were published, the percentage of good results has decreased, this being found even sometimes by the same author (Maher). In the earliest studies the percentage of good results is 75 to 80% (Maher in his first series; Brown) while in later studies (Tank *et al.* 1963; Mark *et al.* 1962, Kennedy *et al.* 1963, Papo *et al.* 1968, Evans *et al.* 1972, Stovner and Endresen 1972, Papo and Visca 1973) good results were obtained in only 35 to 50%.

In our series of 37 patients who underwent phenol injections for *pain of cancerous origin* we have summarized our results as good in cases where analgesic medication could be totally withheld for at least a month or until death, satisfactory when medication could be reduced only partially, and unsatisfactory when pain was not modified by phenolization.

Thus, we obtained 7 good results (41%), 5 satisfactory or incomplete results (29%) and 5 failures (30%) in 17 cases of brachial or cervical pain. In 7 cases of thoraco-abdominal pain we obtained 6 good results (85%) and in 13 cases of lower abdominal, pelvic or inferior limb pain good results were obtained in 53% of the cases, and satisfactory or incomplete results in 23%.

These results must be considered in the light of the general state of the pa-

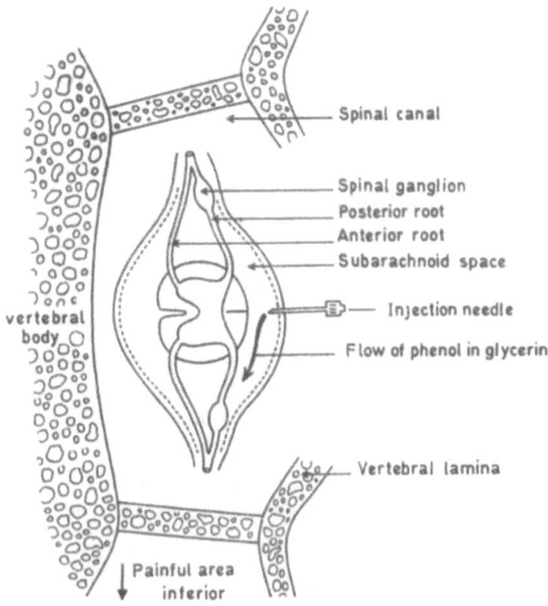

Fig. 9. Placement of lumbar puncture needle for phenol injection

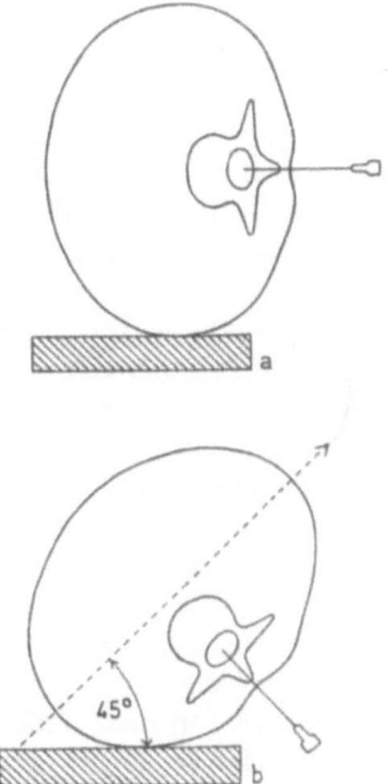

Fig. 10. Phenolization: a) initial position for lumbar puncture, b) position during injection, patient leening 45° backwards

tients, who had advanced cancer which precluded any curative therapy. The survival of our patients was 8 months in the best cases, but only 3 weeks in the most serious ones. There was a 25 to 30% failure rate, even after repeated phenolizations, which we performed in approximately one-third of our patients. These results correspond with those found in the most recent and detailed studies.

From the experience gained till now, chemical rhizotomy appears to give very good results in thoraco-abdominal pain where a relatively large quantity of a concentrated phenol solution can be used (2 to 3 ml of 7.5 to 10% solution); good results are obtained in almost two-thirds of such cases.

Pelvic, recto-vaginal and lower limb pain are also very good indications for this technique, it is even the treatment of choice in patients where the pain is bilateral and where a poor general state as well as a limited life expectancy are contra-indications for even percutaneous cordotomy. The chances of success are great (more than 50 to 60% chance of success) but possible sphincter complications must be borne in mind.

On the contrary we obtained good results in only 40% of our patients who had pain involving the brachial plexus, and in particular, in cases of Pancoast's Syndrome; these results, which are not very satisfying are in line with those of other authors who are unanimous in pointing out the numerous failures and early recurrences in such cases. Maher already pointed out in his first publications the large number of failures, which he attributed to the tendency of pulmonary neoplasm to quickly invade the spinal cord and roots, forming a neoplastic layer which hinders the action of the phenol (Maher 1957, Brown 1958, Mark *et al.* 1962). In addition, at this level the nerve roots have a very short intra-thecal course which limits the effect of the phenol.

However, tumoral involvement of the nerve roots is not the only reason to explain all of the failures of the method and psychological factors must certainly be considered (Stovner and Endresen 1972)—among others, the degree of "cerebral pain fixation" and the extent of the patient's dependence on ever more powerful analgesic drugs.

As a general rule, the method is very useful for thoracic, thoraco-abdominal, rectal and perineal pain where it is easily possible to obtain good results in more than 50% of cases. The method is less useful in upper limb pain where the failure rate can easily be as much as 60 to 75% depending upon which series is analyzed. In such instances, it can only be used as a last resort in certain, carefully defined cases. Crural pain does not lend itself to treatment by this method since percutaneous cordotomy is always preferred.

The failure rate in cases of long lasting cancer pain is close to the failure rate which occurs when phenolization is used for *pain syndromes of a non-neoplastic origin.* Maher had already raised this problem and quickly pointed out that phenol relieves only continuous, relatively well limited pain of cancerous origin as opposed to the acute pain of a fracture or of vertebral lesions where pains were widely distributed.

We have performed one or more phenolizations in 11 cases of "benign pain". Three cases of thoraco-abdominal pain were treated, all of them ending in failure, even though in two of the cases the pain was reduced for approximately one week. Seven cases of costo-pleural pain secondary to existing empyemas, surgical scars

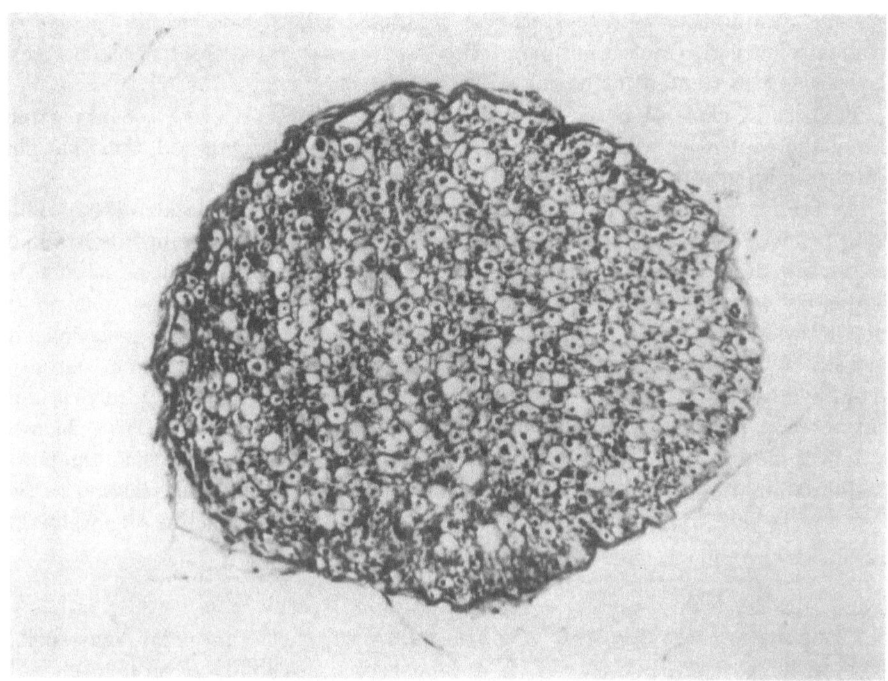

Fig. 11. Demyelinisation of a posterior root after injection of a phenol solution (Holmes silver staining)

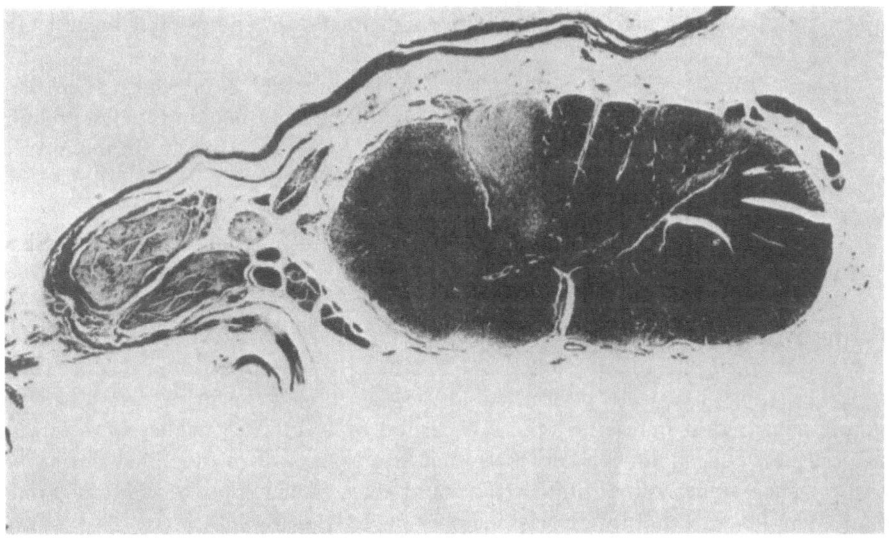

Fig. 12. Demyelinisation of roots end one of the posteriors columns after injection of a phenol solution (Luxol fast blue)

or costal granulomas were treated with 5 failures and 2 good results (sequels of purulent pleurisy). One case of pain following traumatic stretching of the brachial plexus was also treated, without the least effect.

Failures in cases of post-zoster pain are not surprising when the important role of the central nervous system in such pain is recalled and the fact that the spinal ganglia generally escape the effect of phenol.

As far as other types of "benign" pain are concerned, Maher (1960, 1963, 1966) believes that these pains are transmitted by rapid conducting fibers which are overall more resistant to the action of phenol. This hypothesis cannot be completely correct because it is sometimes possible to have persistent pain in an anesthetized territory. In effect, there is a purely quantitative relationship between the sensory deficit and the therapeutic effect. This statement can also be applied to cases of pain recurrence since it is known, by autopsy verification, that there is no regeneration of the damaged fibers. Papo *et al.* (1973) believe that it is necessary to invoke a central, medullary factor and that temporo-spatial summation mechanisms must be foreseen at this level and related to the effects of facilitation of stimuli in the spinal cord, in line with the hypothesis of Melzack and Wall.

4. Complications

Complications are relatively rare and unimportant, the principal cause being errors in the technique employed. If the theoretical possibility of an intra-medullary injection is not considered, the sequelae are infrequent and short lasting if the previously explained rules of technique are followed. These rules deal with the placement of the needle, the quantity and the concentration of the substance injected and especially to accept a compromise between the desired benefit and a certain risk of morbidity.

This is true in cases of cervical and cervico-brachial pain where there is a risk of headaches and a meningeal syndrome, which may be troublesome, due to the proximity of the posterior fossa. It is also true in cases of pain involving the last roots of the cauda equina where pain relief is obtained, occasionally, at the price of urinary incontinence.

A meningeal syndrome often occurs during the first few hours after phenolization performed above the Th 6 level, even more so because at the thoracic and cervico-thoracic levels a larger amount (1.5 to 2 ml) and higher concentration (7.5 rather than 5%) of solution is often used. This meningeal syndrome can be very severe (7 of our 48 injections), but fortunately it lasts for only a short time.

When injections were performed above the Th 6 level other troubles were almost constant in our series; these consisted of headaches, which were serious on occasion, and slight neck stiffness, but the temperature remained normal as a rule. The cerebro-spinal fluid was normal most of the time, or contained only a few lymphocytes (habitually less than 10 per ml).

The seriousness of this syndrome could be reduced by proper positioning of the patient and by keeping the patient in the same position for at least 4 hours after the injection was performed. It is especially important to keep the patient's head in a raised position when he is returned to his bed. We have also systematically avoided performing any injections above the C 5—C 6 level.

Hypotension, sometimes pronounced, can be seen after injection in the cervico-dorsal or high dorsal level; it is probably related to damage to the radicular sympathetic components. It is often of a short duration and never requires any specific therapy. The rate of its occurrence is also very difficult to determine exactly; we have seen it clearly manifested three times, in 24 cases of phenolization between C 6—C 7 and Th 2—Th 3; Papo *et al.* (1968) have already pointed out the existence of this complication.

Sphincter problems, characterized by retention or incontinence, are not rare when a phenol solution is injected below the L 4 level. It probably constitutes the principal complication of phenolization of the posterior roots, in view of the special place that lumbo-sacral and sacral pain occupies among the indications for this technique. However, according to many authors such effects are often transitory and their occurrence is relatively low.

In our 11 cases of lower lumbar or lumbo-sacral phenolization, we had 3 cases of lasting sphincter problems but all of these regressed after several weeks. It should be pointed out that bilateral injections were performed in two of these cases. Our results are similar to those found in larger series (Maher 1955, Nathan and Scott 1958, Tank *et al.* 1963, Papo, Visca, and Caruselli 1968, White and Sweet 1969, Flanigan and Boof 1974).

Sphincter problems must be considered as of little importance, especially in cases of single injections for unilateral pain. However, if a bilateral lumbo-sacral block is to be performed, the risk of sphincter problems is certainly high, although difficult to exactly quantify, but it is avoidable if the analgesic block is performed in two different sessions. For this reason we do not think that bilateral phenolization for intense bilateral pelvic or lumbo-sacral pain must be reserved only for patients with pre-existing bladder and rectal problems.

Paretic problems of the limbs, as a sequel of phenolization, are rare in cases of upper limb pain because the sensory and motor roots are separated at this level and a selective lesion of the posterior roots is easy to perform. In comparison, motor injury is almost inevitable in cases of injection for pain concerning the lumbar dermatomes.

In 6 cases of crural pain of cancerous origin, 3 had lasting paretic sequels of the thigh and leg. This paretic complication, due to the injection level, is almost inevitable and is related to the anatomical impossibility of separating the anterior and posterior roots from contact with the neurotoxic solution. Several authors (Tank *et al.* 1963, Flanigan and Boof 1974, Evans and Mackay 1972) have pointed out this particularly serious and frequent complication which constitutes a contra-indication of the method for crural pain (Papo *et al.* 1968). In such cases, it is preferable to perform a percutaneous cordotomy, especially if the patient is in a good general state and has a presumably long life expectancy.

Other, even rarer complications have been reported and should be considered as exceptional accidents. Smiths (1964) reported a case of fatal meningitis two days after the injection of phenol mixed with silver nitrate. He did not specify if it was a bacterial infection but simply pointed out in this case the presence of lepto-meningitis below the C 8 medullary level and recalled the absence of medullary lesions in 19 autopsied cases reported in the literature.

In 1970 Hughes reported a case of medullary infarction at Th 5 by thrombosis of the posterior spinal arteries after phenolization.

Superville-Sovak *et al.* in 1975 reported 1 patient who had a respiratory arrest and died 5 weeks after the injection of 3 ml of 6% phenol in glycerin. Cerebellar infarction and extended thickening of the cervical, medullary and cerebellar lepto-meninges was found. These accidents are exceptions which remind us of the necessity of fundamental precautions based upon a meticulous puncture technique and the injection of measured quantities of solutions. Thus, White and Sweet (1969) believe that these risks are practically non-existent if the technique is closely followed.

IV. Conclusion

Although the original hypothesis of a specific action of neurolytic agents on afferent fibers conducting pain has never been verified anatomically, in spite of the clinical and even electrophysiological arguments in its favor (at least for the acute phase), the sub-arachnoid injection of alcohol, or particularly phenol, is a useful analgesic tool.

The method is simple, effective and without any great danger, especially if a hyperbaric solution of phenol dissolved in glycerin is used. This is more easily manipulated than alcohol which is hypobaric and, because of this, its diffusion is more difficult to control.

As long as one has acquired enough experience with the method, it is a simple and rapid treatment for pain, easily accepted by the patient, thanks to the speed with which it is performed and to its non-surgical character. It is especially indicated for pain of cancerous origin in patients whose poor general state is a contra-indication for any more extensive neurosurgical procedures. At the present time, the method is in competition with percutaneous cordotomy.

One may confidently expect good results in at least 50%; the average of different studies reported in the literature reaches 60% of good results, especially in cases of pain involving the inferior half of the body. It is in these cases that the technique of intra-thecal phenolization had reduced the indications for open antero-lateral cordotomy by 50% (White and Sweet 1969). However as Papo *et al.* stated, it is very difficult to determine an exact percentage of good results and each case must be considered separately, with regard to the patient's general state, the degree of tumor extension and the individual life expectancy.

In course of time, the use of chemical rhizotomy varied in relation with the development of pain therapy and it may be asked what will be its future. At present, percutaneous antero-lateral cordotomy competes with it, seeing that both techniques are not surgical and well supported by the patients. Nevertheless chemical rhizotomy is still very useful in case of bilateral pelvic and lower limb pain syndromes or when the pain is well circumscribed to a limited area. We do not know wether the percutaneous radiofrequency rhizotomy (Uematsu *et al.* 1974) whose results deserve further experience is a worthwhile method. Thanks to the microscope, surgical rhizotomy has regained interest during these two last years because of the possibility of selective section of posterior radices which conduct pain (Sindou *et al.* 1974, Vlahovitch and Fuentes 1975) but this surgical technique is indicated for long-lasting and limited pain syndromes. Finally, we are of the opinion that chemical rhizotomy by intrathecal injection keeps its place in the field of treatment of pain, providing a meticulous technique and a judicious selection of cases.

References

Abbott, W. D., 1936: Intraspinal injection of absolute alcohol for intractable pain. Amer. J. Surg. *31*, 351—353.

Adson, A. W., 1937: The value of and indications for intraspinal injections of alcohol in the relief of pain. Minn. Med. *20*, 135—140.

Andre-Balisaux, G., Gonsette, R., 1963: Etude anatomo-pathologique des effets de la phénolisation au niveau des cônes terminaux et des racines de la queue de cheval. Acta neurol. belg. *63*, 489—498.

Ansbro, F. P., 1950: Intraspinal segmental alcohol block for relief of intractable pain. Amer. J. Surg. *79*, 276—281.

Baxter, D. W., Schacherl, V., 1962: Experimental studies on the morphological changes produced by intrathecal phenol. Canad. Med. Ass. J. *86/26*, 1200—1205.

Berry, K., Olszewski, J., 1963: Pathology of intrathecal phenol injection in man. Neurology *13*, 152—154.

Bonica, J. J., 1954: The management of pain. Philadelphia: Lea Febiger.

Bradford, F. K., 1959: The use of a caudal air bubble in the control of alcohol injection to relieve flexion reflexes. J. Neurosurg. *16*, 468—470.

Brihaye, J., Retif, J., Gregoire, A., 1961: L'injection sous-arachnoïdienne d'alcool dans le traitement de la douleur. Communication au Congrès International d'Anesthésiologie. Namur.

— — — 1962: Le traitement chirurgical de la douleur. Acta chir. belg., suppl. II — 253—476, pp. 296—307.

Brown, A. S., 1958: Treatment of intractable pain by subarachnoid injection of carbolic acid. Lancet *2*, 975—978.

Coggeshall, R. E., Applebaum, M. L., Fazen, M., Stubbs, T. B., Sykes, M. T., 1975: Unmyelinated axons in human ventral roots, a possible explanation for the failure of dorsal rhizotomy to relieve pain. Brain *98*, 157—166.

Cooper, I. S., Hirose, T., Matsuoka, S., Roth, D., Waltz, J. M., Ericsson, A. D., 1965: Specific neurotoxic perfusion: a new approach to selected cases of pain and spasticity. Neurology *15*, 985—993.

De Bisschop, G., Dumoulin, J., 1967: A propos du garrot ischémique. Electrodiagnostic *4*, 75—81.

De Jesus, P. V., Jr., Hausmanowa-Petrusewicz, I., Barchi, R. L., 1973: The effect of cold on nerve conduction of human slow and fast nerve fibers. Neurology *23*, 1182—1189.

Derrick, W. S., 1970: Control of pain in the cancer patient by subarachnoid alcohol block. Postgraduate Medicine *48*, 232—237.

Dogliotti, A. M., 1931: Traitement des syndromes douloureux de la périphérie par l'alcoolisation sous-arachnoïdienne des racines postérieures à leur émergence de la moelle épinière. Presse Méd. *39*, 1249—1252.

— 1943: Indikationen und Resultate der subarachnoïdalen Alkoholisation der Rückenmarkswurzeln. Wien. Med. Wschr. *18—19*, 295—298.

— 1957: Méthodes chirurgicales périphériques pour le traitement de la douleur chez les cancéreux. Rapports du XVIIe Congrès Soc. Int. Chir. Mexico.

Dunphy, J. E., Alt, R. E., 1936: The relief of pain by the subarachnoid injection of alcohol. The New England J. Med. *214*, 472—477.

Evans, R. J., Mackay, I. M., 1972: Subarachnoid phenol nerve blocks for relief of pain in advanced malignancy. Canad. J. Surg. *15*, 50—53.

Flanigan, S., Boop, W. C., 1974: Spinal intrathecal injection procedures in the management of pain. Clin. Neurosurg. *21*, 229—238.

Gallager, H. S., Yonezawa, T., Hay, R. C., Derrick, W., 1961: Subarachnoid alcohol block. II. Histologic changes in the central nervous system. Amer. J. Path. *38*, 679—693.

Gasser, H. S., Erlanger, J., 1929: The role of fiber size in the establishment of a nerve block by pressure of cocaine. Amer. J. Physiol. *88*, 581—591.

Gillman, J., 1972: Pain relief and other effects following barbotage. Lancet *1*, 746.

Goff, C. W., 1936: Sciatic neuralgia controlled by intraspinal (subarachnoid) injections of ethyl alcohol. Amer. J. Surg. *32*, 37.

Groff, R. A., 1939: Alcoholic injections for the relief of intractable pain. Surg. Clin. N. Amer. *19*, 1569—1581.

— Lewy, F. H., 1941: Dangers of subarachnoid injection of alcohol for relief of pain. Arch. Neurol. Psych. *45*, 533—535.

Grant, F. C., 1941: Surgical methods for the relief of pain. J. A. M. A. *116*, 567—571.

Greenhill, J. P., Schmitz, H. E., 1935: Intraspinal (subarachnoid) injection of alcohol for pain associated with malignant conditions of the female genitalia. J. A. M. A. *105*, 406—409.

Guttman, S. A., Pardee, I., 1944: Spinal cord level syndrome following intrathecal ammonium sulfate and procaine hydrochloride. A case report with autopsy findings. Anesthesiology *5*, 347—353.

Hand, L. V., 1944: Subarachnoid ammonium sulfate therapy for intractable pain. Anesthesiology *5*, 354—358.

Hansebout, R. R., Cosgrove, J. B. R., 1966: Effects of intrathecal phenol in man. Neurology *16*, 277—282.

Hariga, J., 1966: Influences sur la motricité de la suppression des effecteurs gamma par alcoolisation des nerfs périphériques. Etude expérimentale chez le chat décérébré. Résultats thérapeutiques dans l'infirmité motrice cérébrale. Acta Neurol. Psych. Belg. *66*, 607—711.

— Tardieu, G., Tardieu, C., Gagnard, L., 1966: Effets de l'application d'alcool dilué sur le nerf. Partie 1: confrontation de l'étude dynamographique et de l'étude histologique chez le chat décérébré. J. Neurol. Sci. *3*, 284—299.

Hay, R. C., Yonezawa, T., Derrick, W. S., 1959: Control of intractable pain in advanced cancer by subarachnoid alcohol block. J. A. M. A. *169*, 1315—1320.

Hitchcock, E., 1969: Osmolytic neurolysis for intractable facial pain. Lancet *1*, 434—436.

Hughes, J. T., 1966: Pathological findings following the intrathecal injection of ethyl alcohol in man. Paraplegia *4*, 167—175.

— 1970: Thrombosis of the posterior spinal arteries: a complication of an intrathecal injection of phenol. Neurology *20*, 659—664.

Iggo, A., Walsh, E. G., 1960: Selective block of small fibres in the spinal roots by phenol. Brain *83*, 701—708.

Kennedy, W. F., Akamatsu, T., 1963: Subarachnoid block with phenol-glycerine for the relief of intractable pain. Anesthesiology *24*, 584—585.

Knott, L. W., Katz, J., Rubinstein, L. J., 1969: Separate and combined effects of phenol, hyaluronidase and dimethyl sulfoxide on the sciatic nerve of the rat. II. Chronic studies. Neurology *19*, 946—953.

Kuzucu, E. Y., Derrick, W. S., Wilber, S. A., 1966: Control of intractable pain with subarachnoid alcohol block. J. A. M. A. *195*, 541—544.

Lourie, H., Vanasupa, P., 1963: Comments on the use of intraspinal phenolpantopaque for relief of pain and spasticity. J. Neurosurg. *20*, 60—63.

Lucas, J. T., Ducker, T. B., Perot, P. L., Jr., 1975: Adverse reactions to intrathecal saline injection for control of pain. J. Neurosurg. *42*, 557—561.

Maher, R. M., 1955. Relief of pain in incurable cancer. Lancet *1*, 18—20.

— 1957: Neurone selection in relief of pain. Further experiences with intrathecal injections. The Lancet *1*, 16—19.

— 1960: Further experiences with intrathecal and subdural phenol. Observations on two forms of pain. The Lancet, 895—899.

Maher, R. M., 1963: Intrathecal chlorocresol in the treatment of pain in cancer. The Lancet *1*, 965—967.

Mark, V. H., White, J. C., Zervas, N. T., Ervin, F. R., Richardson, E. P., 1963: Intrathecal use of phenol for the relief of chronic severe pain. New Engl. J. Med. *267*, 589—593.

Nathan, P. W., 1959: Intrathecal phenol to relieve spasticity in paraplegia. The Lancet *II*, 1099—1102.

— Scott, T. G., 1958: Intrathecal phenol for intractable pain: safety and dangers of method. Lancet *1*, 76—80.

— Sears, T. A., 1960: Effects of phenol on nervous conduction. J. Physiol. *150*, 565—580.

— — Smith, M. C., 1965: Effects of phenol solutions on the nerve roots of the cat: an electrophysiological and histological study. J. Neurol. Sci. *2*, 7—29.

Olmsted, J. M. D., Hodgson, P., 1931: An explanation of the results of the "alcohol block". Amer. J. Physiol. *97*, 597—601.

Ottley, C., 1938: Intrathecal alcohol injection for relief of pain: a review. Brit. Med. J. 510—512.

Papo, I., Visca, A., Caruselli, G., 1968: Indications et limites de la radicotomie chimique par le phénol sous-arachnoïdien dans le traitement des algies cancéreuses. Neurochirurgie *14*, 617—626.

— Pellegrini, G., Scarlato, G., 1967: La radicotomie chimique par substances phénoliques. Acta Neurol. Psychiat. Belg. *67*, 125—132.

— Visca, A., 1973: Intrathecal phenol in the treatment of cancer pain. J. Neurosurg. Sci. *17*, 146—156.

Pedersen, E., Reske-Nielsen, E., 1965: Neuropathology of subarachnoid phenol-glycerin. Acta Neuropathol. *5*, 112—116.

Peyton, W. T., Semansky, E. J., Baker, A. B., 1937: Subarachnoid injection of alcohol for relief of intractable pain with discussion of cord changes found at autopsy. Amer. J. Cancer *30*, 709—717.

Pitts, W., Browder, J., 1939: Spinal subarachnoid injection of absolute alcohol for the relief of intractable pain. Ann. Surg. *109*, 33—42.

Poppen, J. L., 1936: The relief of pain by the use of subarachnoid alcohol injection. Indications, contra-indications, technics and results in 82 patients. Surg. Clin. N. Amer. *16*, 1663—1668.

Rasminsky, M., 1973: The effects of temperature on conduction in demyelinated single nerve fibers. Arch. Neurol. *28*, 287—292.

Russell, W. R., 1936: Intraspinal injection of alcohol for intractable pain. Lancet *1*, 595—599.

Saltzstein, H. C., 1934: Intraspinal (subarachnoid) injection of absolute alcohol: for the control of pain in far advanced malignant growths. J. A. M. A. *103*, 242—243.

Savitz, M. H., Malis, L. I., 1973: Intractable pain treated with intrathecal isotonic iced saline. J. Neurol. Neurosurg. Psychiat. *36*, 417—420.

Schaumburg, H., Byck, R., Herman, R., Rosengart, C., 1967: Peripheral nerve damage by cold. Arch. Neurol. *16*, 103—109.

Schaumburg, H. H., Byck, R., Weller, R. O., 1970: The effect of phenol on peripheral nerve; an histological and electrophysiological study. J. Neuropath. Exp. Neurol. *29*, 615—630.

Sindou, M., Fischer, G., Goutelle, A., Mansuy, L., 1974: La radicellotomie postérieure sélective. Premiers résultats dans la chirurgie de la douleur. Neurochirurgie *20*, 391—408.

Sloane, P., 1935: Syndrome referable to the cauda equina following the intraspinal injection of alcohol for relief from pain. Arch. Neurol. Psych. *34*, 1120—1123.

Smith, M. C., 1964: Histological findings following intrathecal injections of phenol solutions for relief of pain. Brit. J. Anaesth. *36*, 387—406.

Stern, E. L., 1934: Relief of intractable pain by the intraspinal (subarachnoid) injection of alcohol. Amer. J. Surg. *25*, 211—227.

Stern, E. L., 1936: The intraspinal injection of alcohol for the relief of pain and for sympathetic nervous system disorders. Med. Rec. *143*, 327—331.

Stewart, W. A., Lourie, H., 1963: An experimental evaluation of the effects of subarachnoid injection of phenol pantopaque in Cats. J. Neurosurg. *20*, 64—72.

Stovner, J., Endresen, R., 1972: Intrathecal phenol for cancer pain. Acta anaesth. Scand. *16*, 17—21.

Superville-Sovak, B., Rasminsky, M., Finlayson, M. H., 1975: Complications of phenol neurolysis. Arch. Neurol. *32*, 226—228.

Tank, T. M., Dohn, D. F., Gardner, W. J., 1963: Intrathecal injections of alcohol or phenol for relief of intractable pain. Cleveland Clin. Quart. *30*, 111—117.

Tardieu, G., Hariga, J., Tardieu, C., Gagnard, L., Velin, J., 1964: Traitement de la spasticité par infiltration d'alcool dilué au point moteur ou par injection épidurale. Rev. Neurol. *110*, 563—565.

— Tardieu, C., Hariga, J., 1971: Infiltrations par alcool à 45° des points moteurs, des racines par voie épidurale, ou du nerf postérieur. Leurs indications et contre-indications dans les divers modes de „spasticité" (expérience de 10 ans). Rev. Neurol. *125*, 63—69.

Todd, T. F., 1939: Relief of intractable pain in carcinoma of the cervix uteri. Lancet *2*, 1305—1308.

Truelsen, F., 1943: Subarachnoid alcohol injection for the relief of intractable pain. Acta Chir. Scand. *88*, 17—32.

Uematsu, S., Udvarhelyi, G. B., Benson, D. W., Siebens, A. A., 1974: Percutaneous radiofrequency rhizotomy. Sur. Neurol. *2*, 319—325.

Vlahovitch, B., Fuentes, J. M., 1975: Résultats de la radicellotomie sélective postérieure à l'étage lombaire et cervical. Neurochirurgie *21*, 29—42.

White, J. C., Sweet, W. H., 1969: Pain and Neurosurgeon. Subarachnoid block with Phenol, pp. 160—167. Springfield, Ill.: Ch. C Thomas.

White, J. C., 1965: Relief of pain in terminal cancer. Surg. Gyn. Obstet. *120*, 115—116.

Zuzucu, E. Y., Derrick, W. S., Wilber, S. A., 1966: Control of intractable pain with subarachnoid alcohol block. J. A. M. A. *195*, 541—544.

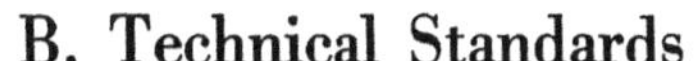

B. Technical Standards

Olfactory Groove and Suprasellar Meningiomas

L. Symon

The Department of Neurosurgical Studies, Institute of Neurology,
The National Hospital, London (England)

With 12 Figures

Contents

Introduction

Meningiomas of the central subfrontal region originating either from the olfactory groove, planum or jugum sphenoidale or suprasellar area, account for about 10% of all meningiomas in a review of the world literature (Cushing and Eisenhardt 1938, Ehlers and Malmros 1973, Fusek and Kunc 1969, Guillaumat 1937, Olivecrona 1967, Zülch 1956), and they are therefore relatively uncommon lesions in general neurosurgical practice. Close association with clinics of ophthalmology, however, increases the referral rate of these interesting lesions. As in most meningiomas, a number of terms have been used to describe their site of origin. The general term, subfrontal, is often regarded as synonomous with the meningiomas arising from the olfactory groove; where the origin can be specified as from the planum or jugum of the sphenoid bone, these sites may be specified; meningiomas arising from one anterior clinoid may be described; and meningiomas arising from the dorsum sellae or from the diaphragma sellae constitute the true suprasellar meningiomas. This paper will deal, in the main, with those arising from the olfactory groove and from the jugum sphenoidale (tuberculum sellae) or from a mixture of the two, and while the latter group are frequently termed suprasellar meningiomas, the author prefers the term "meningioma of the jugum sphenoidale" since that more nearly describes their site of origin. As in most meningiomas, the attribution of a primary site of origin to a large tumour may be extremely difficult, and while these two main groups—the olfactory groove and the jugum tumours—tend to run true to type, extension laterally along the sphenoidal wing does occur from time to time, thereby increasing the difficulty of classification and also, incidentally, the difficulties of removal of the tumour.

This paper will divide these tumours from the operative point of view into two groups: the true meningioma of the planum or jugum sphenoidale, and those of the olfactory groove, bearing in mind that specific difficulties of technique applicable to either may arise in a large tumour which has spread from one site to involve the other as well.

The Presenting Features of Meningiomas of the Olfactory Groove and Jugum Sphenoidale

The dominant features in the clinical presentation of these masses are three: visual field defects, epilepsy, and psychological change. Epilepsy in these lesions is of grand mal type and, when it occurs, is almost invariably the first noticed feature. It is much commoner in meningiomas of the olfactory groove and, indeed, rare in more posteriorly placed lesions, but the incidence in olfactory groove tumours of 30% in the author's series is appreciably lower than the often quoted 50% incidence in meningiomas generally, and of value only since it may draw the attention of the patient to an otherwise completely silent mass.

Psychological changes occur predominantly in olfactory groove tumours also, since particularly those which do not include epilepsy in their development may reach a large size before signs of raised intracranial pressure or eventual encroachment on the optic pathways bring the patient to surgery. Minor psychological changes are frequently observed, taking the form of loss of memory or confusion, while dementia, euphoria or antisocial behaviour present in at least subtle form on enquiry in about half of current cases. More obtrusive psychological change is relatively rare and confined almost exclusively to large, subfrontal masses. Two cases in the author's experience have presented with personality deterioration so severe as to occasion divorce, happily remarriage (to the same partner) being a feature of the post-operative course in one of them.

In both olfactory groove and suprasellar meningiomas, the commonest presenting feature is impairment of visual function. In olfactory groove tumours this invariably indicates a very large lesion which has extended backwards to embarrass the chiasmal structures from their upper aspect, but in tumours arising directly from the jugum sphenoidale or from the anterior clinoidal area, visual impairment is often an early sign. Regrettably, since the visual impairment frequently manifests itself in one eye very much earlier than the other, the sinister nature of the visual loss is often unrecognised and a considerable time may pass between the onset of visual symptoms and the submission of the patient to investigation and surgery. In 40 current cases, visual embarrassment was absent in only six; in both olfactory groove and jugum lesions the visual loss was generally bilateral but almost invariably more severe in one eye. The classical symmetrical, bitemporal hemianopia of the pituitary mass is less common in this type of lesion, being more usually an asymmetrical hemianopia which is, however, usually temporal in distribution. As in pituitary tumours, however, early embarrassment of the optic pathways frequently presents as a central scotoma, and it is essential therefore that full central field assessment accompany the more straightforward peripheral field mapping in the analysis of these visual defects. Probably the commonest early visual complaint is blurred vision in one eye, usually betokening a central scotoma. Sometimes, indeed, the loss of vision in one eye proceeds almost unnoticed by the patient—one of the author's cases with a very large tumour became aware that one eye was blind only a few weeks before he developed the headaches and vomiting of raised intracranial pressure, when his return to shooting game after an absence of many years required him to close one eye to aim his rifle.

Clinical Examination

Clinical examination of subfrontal meningiomas may frequently reveal no clues other than the visual field defects. These may be accompanied by optic atrophy on one or both sides, or by papilloedema. The classical Foster-Kennedy syndrome with pallor of one optic disc and papilloedema in the other eye is, however, uncommon, being present in only one of the author's 40 cases. Loss or impairment of the sense of smell which might be thought inevitable, particularly with large olfactory groove tumours, is often disappointingly absent. Thus, in eight massive, bilateral olfactory groove tumours filling the entire medial frontal zone bilaterally, no less than four were recorded as having normal sense of smell pre-operatively. In the more posteriorly placed, jugum lesions, some impairment of smell on at least one side may be detected and this, in association with visual defects, should raise the possibility of a specific diagnosis. The common types of olfactory stimulation used clinically, such as cloves and peppermint, have recently been suggested to provide more than true olfactory stimulation, however, and it may be that more subtle testing with strict olfactory stimuli would reveal a higher proportion of reduced olfactory function. Whatever the route of sensation, the preserved detection of odours is usually lost following excision, particularly with large bilateral tumours. Long tract signs—involvement of the pyramidal pathways—are uncommon unless the tumour has reached a very large size.

Investigations

Investigations should be aimed at confirmation of the diagnosis in the first instance and, beyond this, to as full a delineation of the size and extent of the tumour as possible.

Investigations should begin with plain films, EEG and EMI scan.

Plain X-Ray

In careful plain films with A-P and lateral tomograms of the subfrontal area, it is frequently possible to suggest the diagnosis of subfrontal meningioma from the presence of localised bone thickening (Fig. 1). Regrettably, even on high quality screening films, small, subtle hyperstotic changes in the jugum sphenoidale are frequently missed even in the best clinics and, as a screening test for the presence or absence of subfrontal meningioma, plain films cannot be regarded as reliable. However, detailed plain skull films may reveal subtle hyperostoses on anterior clinoid, jugum sphenoidale, or a portion of the olfactory groove. Blistering of the sphenoidal sinus, that is the extension of the sphenoidal sinus in a small curve (Fig. 2) in the base of the meningioma, is another specific feature which may be evident on plain films. In meningiomas of the jugum sphenoidale, a fairly characteristic shortening of the dorsum sellae is often present. While this feature may be insufficient to make certain diagnosis by itself since it occurs with other tumours in the suprasellar region such as craniopharyngioma, in association with subsequent radiological investigations it may prompt a correct pre-operative diagnosis.

EMI Scan

Computerised axial tomography, the most advanced and non-traumatic method of detailed neuroradiological investigation yet available, is of value in the preliminary investigation of any neurosurgical problem but, in small lesions close to the base, its value is possibly less than in most other situations. Thus the differentiation between the jugum itself and a small, suprasellar mass, may prove extremely difficult, although enhancement with Conray and careful attention to repetition of the tomograms at exactly similar levels, may reveal a mass on Conray enhancement which is not present on the plain EMI scan. This, of course, makes the diagnosis of a suprasellar meningioma likely.

With larger olfactory groove or suprasellar masses, the EMI scan will delineate the shape of the mass in a transverse tomographic plane, thus adding to the three-dimensional perspective which the surgeon obtains from AEG and angiography, and considerably easing the planning of surgical excision (Fig. 3).

Electro-Encephalography

The EEG, almost invariably performed in neurosurgical clinics, is abnormal in about two-thirds of subfrontal tumours, particularly those of large size, but the abnormality is not usually specific. It is of no value in localisation and in the planning of surgical treatment.

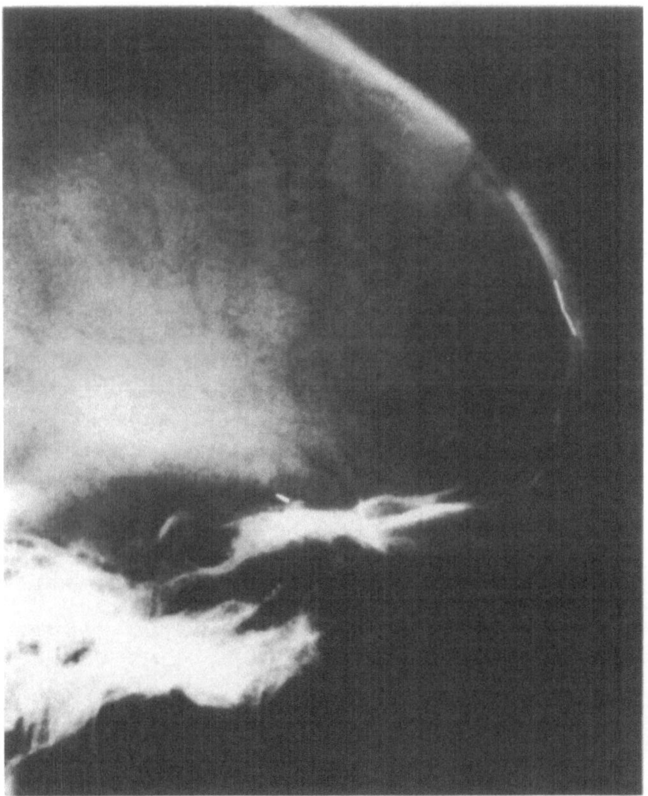

Fig. 1. Post-operative film of a patient after unilateral excision of a meningioma of the jugum sphenoidale. The hyperostosis is shown in the region of a silver clip on the jugum

Gamma Scan

Gamma scan investigation is generally positive in subfrontal tumours if they have reached a size of more than 2 cm in extent (Fig. 4), but small, particularly jugum, masses may well be missed. The uptake of the base of skull may be impossible to differentiate from the uptake of a small suprasellar tumour and a negative gamma scan cannot therefore be regarded as excluding a suprasellar meningioma.

Angiography

Carotid angiography is the single most important investigation in the delineation of olfactory groove and suprasellar tumours. As in neurosurgery generally, many of the difficulties of excision of these tumours arise from their potential involvement with major blood vessels. Thus, in the case of the olfactory groove tumour (Fig. 5), the major portions of the anterior cerebral artery may be closely applied to the postero-superior aspects of the tumour, and may require careful dissection from the capsule in the course of removal. It is, in the author's view,

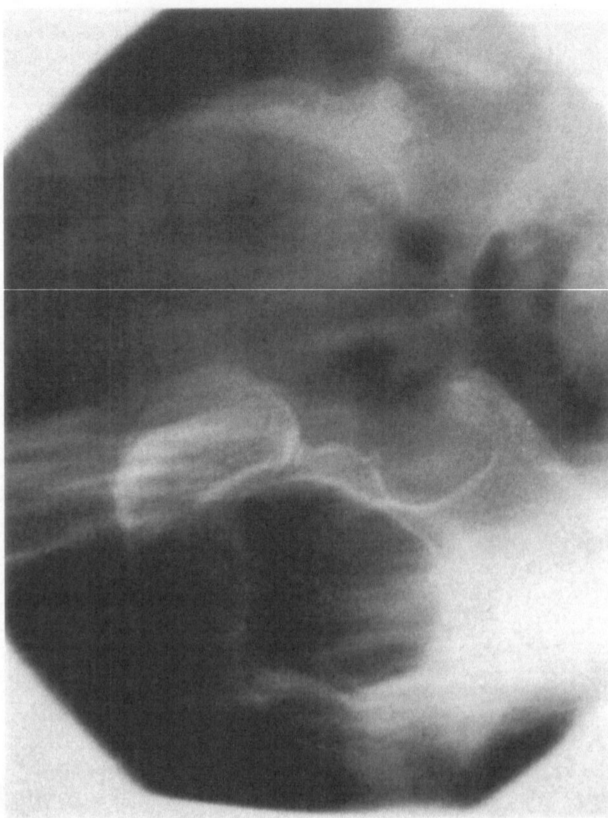

Fig. 2. Midline tomogram (during air encephalography) showing the blistering of the sphenoidal sinus into the bone involved in the base of a meningioma arising from the planum sphenoidale. Calcification in the base of the tumour is also visible, while the extent of the tumour is partially outlined by subfrontal air

essential that those vessels be adequately delineated by angiography pre-operatively. In smaller masses, lesser displacement of subfrontal branches of the anterior cerebral circulation may be revealed with the aid, if necessary, of magnification angiography. The mass itself may show pathological circulation and substraction techniques may greatly enhance the contrast of such pathological circulation, perhaps even completely delineating the size of the mass on A-P and lateral films, and being particularly valuable in demonstrating the major portals of entry of the blood supply. In both olfactory groove and the jugum masses, the arterial supply generally comes from the ophthalmic circulation via ethmodial perforating branches. Particularly where the mass is large and the vascularity considerable, a knowledge of the point of entry of these major vessels is of great use in the course of surgery (Fig. 6). Supplementary blood supply, especially in larger tumours, may arise from branches of the anterior cerebral artery in the capsule, but not infrequently the circulation of the brain itself is completely uninvolved. In this group of tumours, involvement of the terminal carotid artery and proximal anterior and middle cerebral vessels is uncommon unless the mass has a more than usually extensive origin involving the inner third of the sphenoidal wing in addition to a true subfrontal situation.

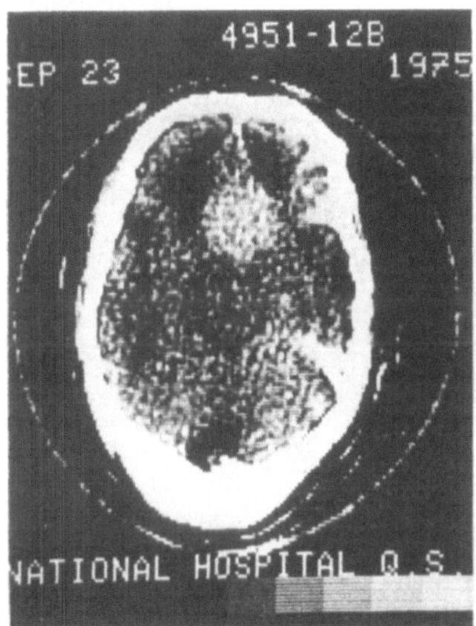

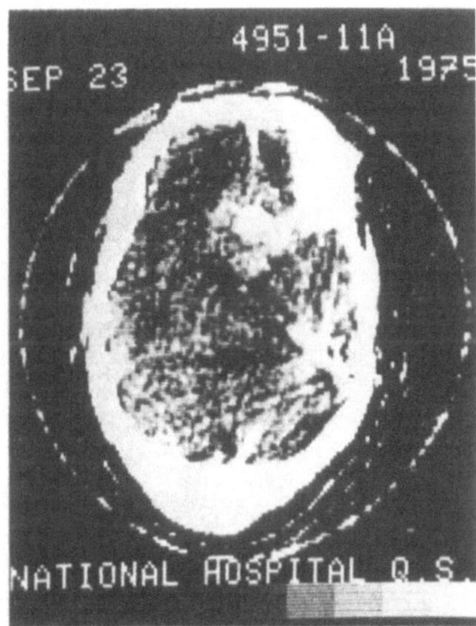

Fig. 3. EMI scans close to the base (11 A) and 1.5 cm above (12 B) in a 74-year-old patient with meningioma of the planum and jugum sphenoidale. The lower cut outlines hyperostosis in the midline in the centre of the meningioma, the upper cut indicates the diameter of the mass. Oedema of both frontal lobes is also evident

Air Encephalography or Ventriculography

In anteriorly placed masses confidently outlined by angiography, preferably with the demonstration of a blush of pathological circulation, visualisation of the mass by air study may be omitted. In the author's view, however, masses on the planum sphenoidale, jugum and suprasellar area, should in addition be outlined by air study either by lumbar route or, in cases with raised intracranial pressure, by ventriculography. The reason for this is that, while a pathological circulation may suggest the size of a suprasellar mass with some confidence and, if this is supported by the computerised axial tomography it may be felt that sufficient information has been obtained, the detailed relationship between the anterior end of the third ventricle, the chiasm, and the top of the tumour, is best demonstrated by AEG. Thus, a certain proportion of jugum sphenoidale tumours take the form of an hour-glass—a portion in front and a portion behind the chiasm. This detail is extremely difficult to elucidate angiographically, but is immediately obvious on AEG or ventriculography. The author's preference is for AEG if

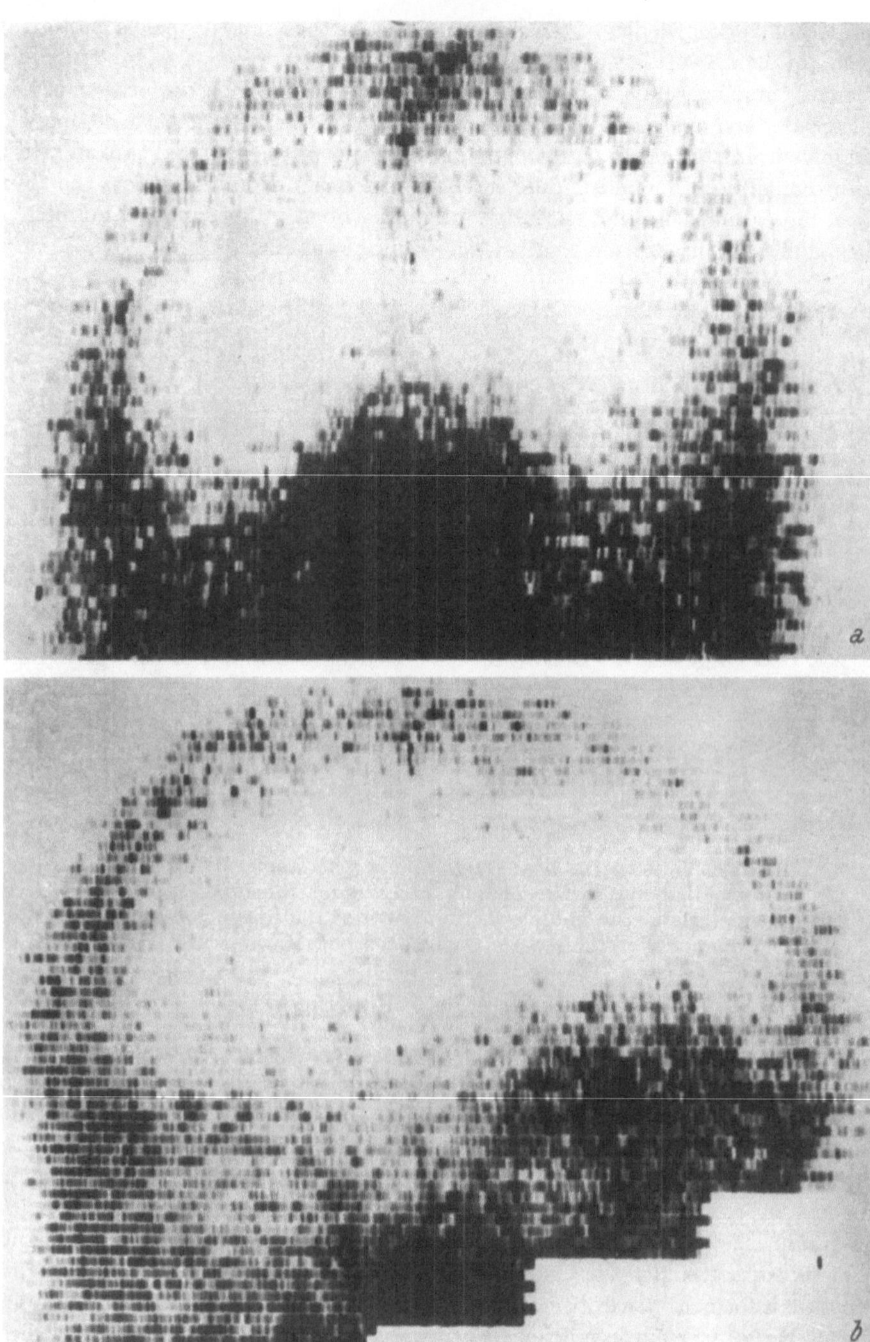

Fig. 4. A-P and lateral views of the gamma scan (Tc 99 m) of a patient with a large olfactory groove and jugum sphenoidale meningioma

possible, since greater delineation of the extent of the tumour in the basal cistern is obtained by A-P and lateral tomography, in addition to clear delineation of the relationship with the anterior end of the third ventricle (Figs. 7 and 8). The considerable operative mortality evident in previous series should convince most surgeons of the possibilities for improvement in the excision of these difficult

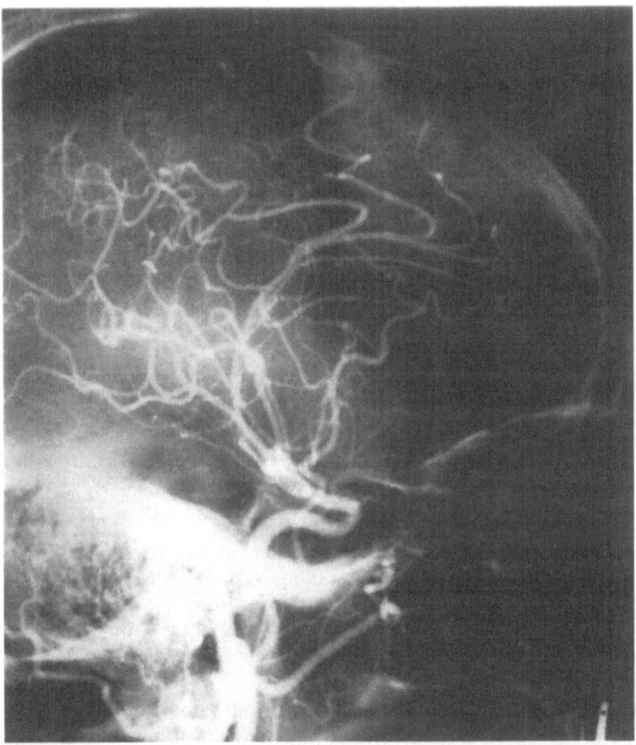

Fig. 5. Lateral view of the carotid angiogram of a large meningioma of the olfactory groove and jugum sphenoidale (bilateral). The relationship of the anterior cerebral arteries to the tumour is clearly outlined, the draping of the peripheral branches of anterior cerebral indicating the anterior margin of the mass

lesions and, in the author's view, a clear image of the potential involvement of suprachiasmal and paraventricular structures in the extent of the tumour is essential in this respect.

Pre-Operative Management

Facilities for adequate blood replacement and the clearance of potential sinus infection is a *sine qua non* of the surgical management of frontal tumours generally, and need scarcely be mentioned. The pre-operative exhibition of dexamethasone may perhaps be less generally accepted but, in the author's experience, dexamethasone in a dosage of 4 mg six-hourly exhibited for 48 hours pre-operatively not only may produce an improvement in visual fields indicating some reduction of size of the mass but also, because of reduction in tissue tension in the mass and adjacent areas, enhances the ease of surgical dissection, and should not be omitted. In the exhibition of dexamethasone, care may be necessary in patients with a history of peptic ulcer but, unless there is evidence that ulceration is currently active, it is the author's practice to exhibit the drug in the belief that the advantages outweigh the potential hazards. The drug may be discontinued gradually from 48 hours post-operatively over a few days.

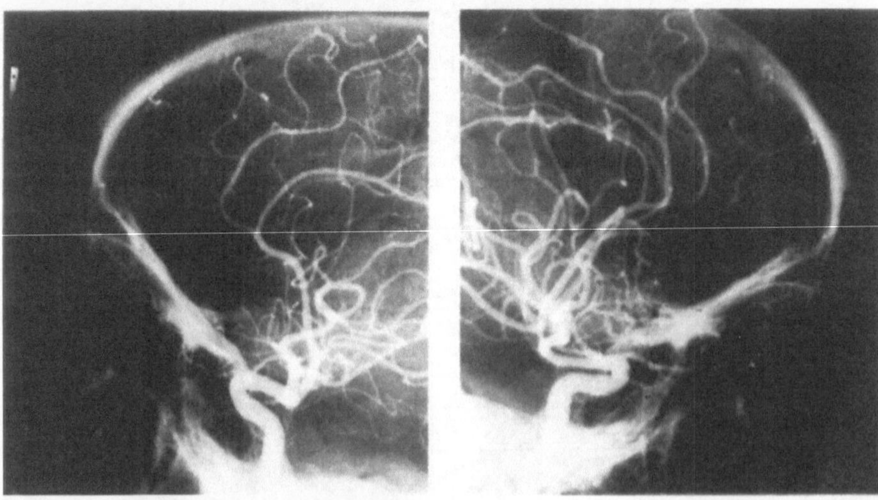

Fig. 6. Lateral views of the right and left carotid arteriogram of a patient with a meningioma of the jugum sphenoidale. The hyperostosis is visible in both lateral views, the pathological circulation of the meningioma itself is partially seen in the right carotid arteriogram, and the ethmoidal arterial supply from the ophthalmic artery is shown in both views, that on the right side being the larger

It is a curious fact that endocrine symptomatology either pre- or post-operatively even in posteriorly placed suprasellar meningiomas, is uncommon. Thus, although the mass may occupy apparently the entire suprasellar area displacing the infundibulum posteriorly and the supra-optic nuclei superiorly, diabetes insipidus is excessively uncommon, having occurred in only one of the author's 40 cases, and evidence of clinical pituitary insufficency is rare. Routine steroid replacement is therefore usually unnecessary. However, in the occasional case where the meningioma transgresses the diaphragma sellae and invades the pituitary fossa itself, particularly where incomplete removal only has been achieved, the possibility of later endocrine involvement from direct destruction of the pituitary should be remembered in management.

Anaesthesia

With lesions such as subfrontal tumours, where access is frequently difficult, it is essential that thought be given to any measures which may render the exposure easier. The use of pre-operative dexamethasone has already been mentioned. The other two chief aids are excellent anaesthesia and adequate positioning of the patient.

The type of anaesthetic used varies widely from one clinic to another, but the anaesthetic colleagues with whom the author has worked for many years have invariably used basic Halothane anaesthesia with controlled ventilation under D-tubocararine, aiming to use a ventilatory volume sufficient to reduce the arterial pCO_2 to the level of around 30 mmHg. A negative phase in ventilation is almost invariably employed, and hypotension achieved either in suitably

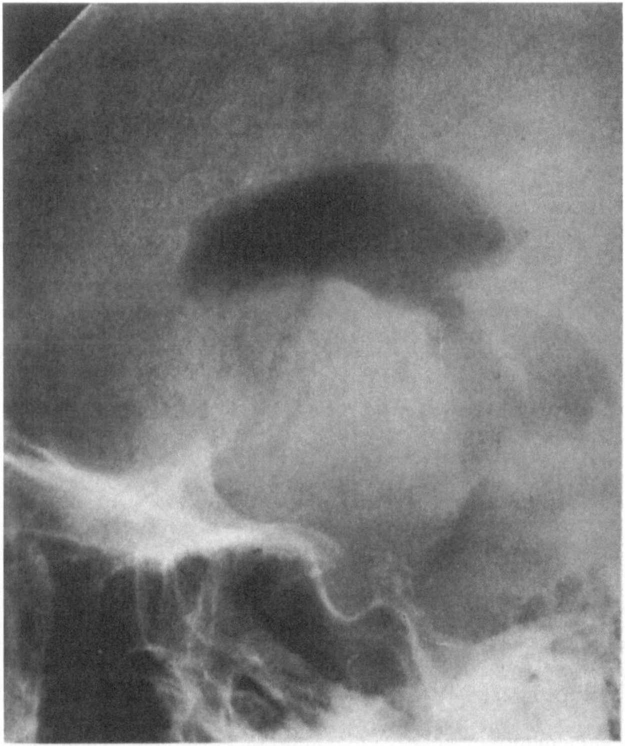

Fig. 7. Lumbar air encephalogram in a large meningioma of the posterior olfactory groove and jugum sphenoidale. The outline of the tumour may be clearly made out in this midline tomogram; its posterior margin overlies the dorsum and extends into the interpeduncular cistern, the 3rd ventricle is rotated backwards, but the direction of its optic recess clearly indicates that the optic nerves are stretched down behind and below the mass

sensitive subjects by a varying Halothane concentration within the limits 0.5 to 1.5% or, in more resistant cases, with the addition of Arfonad (Trimetaphan) as necessary. Deep hypotension is seldom necessary or desirable in the removal of such tumours, but where the anterior ethmoidal supply is profuse, determined reduction of the blood pressure to the level of 60 mmHg systolic may be necessary for some time, to enable difficult dissection down to the blood supply of the tumour to be achieved in the face of profuse haemorrhage. This aspect will be discussed further under "technique".

Control of venous tension is usually achieved satisfactorily by adequate ventilation with a negative phase, but in the case of very large tumours with extremely raised intracranial pressure, the use of intravenous mannitol may have to be considered. This drug, given in a dose of 40 g intravenously fairly rapidly at the time of the induction of anaesthesia, will appreciably reduce intracranial tension by the time the tumour is approached. In subfrontal lesions, the hypervolaemic phase following mannitol infusion does not usually occasion

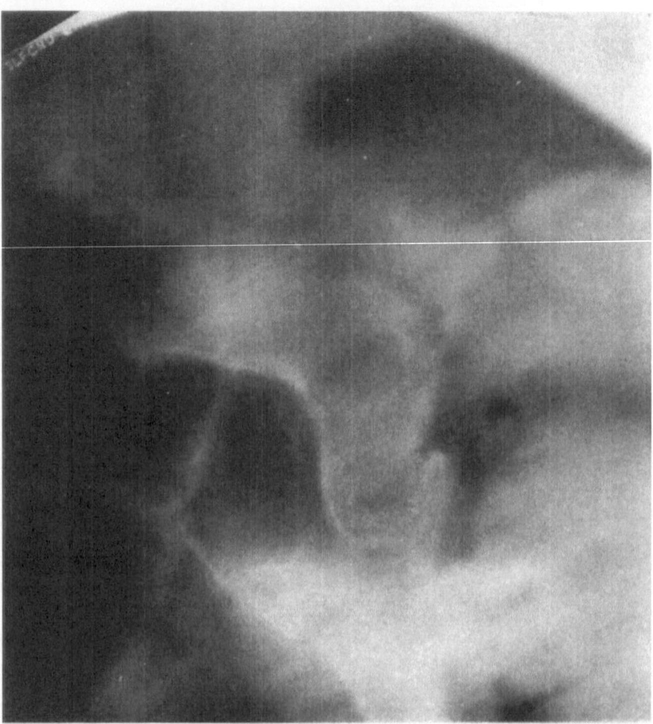

Fig. 8. Air encephalogram in a case of meningioma of the jugum sphenoidale extending into the suprasellar area. The outline of the mass is visible, and the slight backward displacement of the 3rd ventricle indicates the relationship of the optic nerves, which embrace the mass roughly halfway down its posterior circumference

too much blood loss since the blood supply of the tumour is not directly attacked during the approach. It should, however, be remembered that most tumours in the subfrontal situation with extensively raised intracranial pressure will require some brain resection for access during the actual excision, and it is the author's practice therefore usually to defer consideration of mannitol infusion until the dura is exposed, when judicious brain needling will determine the site and depth of the anterior portion of the tumour, and enable planned resection of the frontal lobe. This procedure may be satisfactorily accomplished even in the face of appreciably raised pressure, as will be subsequently described, and may obviate the necessity for mannitol infusion completely. The susceptibility of brain to retraction under mannitol, with the frequently observed fragility of small surface vessels, is therefore avoided.

Positioning the Patient

Head position in the approach to subfrontal tumours represents a compromise. A large subfrontal tumour extending forward to or in front of the crista galli demands, in its most anterior portions, appreciable flexion of the head for ease of surgical access, whilst the posterior and superior portions of the true olfactory groove tumour and the dome of the jugum or suprasellar lesion demand that the head be in neutral or even slightly extended position to facilitate as direct access as possible to the vessels around the top of the olfactory groove mass, or the vessels, chiasm and juxta third-ventricular structures in relation to the apex of the jugum mass. It is occasionally useful, therefore, to change the degree of head extension in the course of the procedure and, if this is not desirable or practicable, to weigh carefully the relative ease of access to these two slightly conflicting demands. The author's general preference is to ensure maximum ease during dissection of the postero-superior portions of these tumours since it is here that the most critical manœuvres are required, and to accept the slight discomfort, bending and peering, necessary to clear the polar portion of an olfactory groove attachment.

Planning the Flap

The first surgical decision necessary in the actual operation is the decision for the type and site of the scalp and bone flap. In general this will depend on the location and size of the tumour, as determined by the pre-operative investigations. Olfactory groove tumours of moderate size whose bulk is equally distributed between right and left sides and almost all tumours of the jugum sphenoidale and suprasellar area are, in the author's view, best approached by a right-sided frontal flap, as indicated in the diagram (Fig. 9a).

A unilateral left-sided flap will be indicated in the rare unilateral olfactory groove tumour well forward on the left side, or in tumours of the olfactory groove which are so asymmetrical that their bulk is vastly predominantly on the left side. Even where an olfactory groove mass of moderate size may be slightly larger on the left, the ease of approach for a right-handed surgeon from the right side, and the fact that the majority of patients are right-handed and that this is therefore the nondominant hemisphere, makes the right-sided approach preferable.

In very large bilateral olfactory groove lesions with extensive involvement of the visual pathways, a bifrontal bone flap may be necessary to enable approach from laterally along the sphenoidal wing on either side, since the mere bulk of tumour may make it impossible to reach the region of the contralateral optic nerve with safety (Fig. 9 c).

A further flap occasionally used by the author is indicated in the diagram (Fig. 9 b). This flap, predominantly right-sided, is carried across the sagittal sinus in its anterior part, and enables division of the sagittal sinus and lateral retraction of the parasagittal frontal lobe on the left side in the case of moderate to large olfactory groove tumours.

The Technique of Excision of Olfactory Groove Meningiomas

Armed with an accurate pre-operative assessment of the size of the tumour and of the likely involvement of the anterior cerebral and terminal carotid vessels, and with an appreciation from the pre-operative ophthalmological assessment of the likely direction of pressure on the optic chiasm, the surgeon will have selected one of the flaps described and will have turned the appropriate bilateral, unilateral or mixed bone flap. He is then faced with a dura whose tension will vary according to the size of the tumour and the excellence of the surgical management to this stage and, except in rare polar extensions of the olfactory groove tumours, he will find no immediate tumour available whose removal will assist in the reduction of intracranial tension.

Uncapping the Tumour

In tumours of the olfactory groove, it is the author's invariable practice to uncap the tumour by a wedge excision of an appropriate piece of frontal lobe on the right side. The extent of this excision is best determined by preliminary brain needling from a point 1½ cm parasagittally and about 1″ to 1½″ behind the pole. The exact posterior distance of the needle track will depend on the site of the maximum height of tumour from the olfactory groove and on the length of the patient's frontal fossa, remembering that wedge excisions should not extend as far posteriorly as the sphenoidal wing, but may generally begin at or just in front of the level of the lateral canthus. Their medial extent should not extend behind the free edge of the falx, and should be planned in relation to the observed displacement of the anterior cerebral circulation. Where the anterior cerebral arteries are tightly applied to the top of a large olfactory groove tumour, it is essential that the wedge excision involve only frontal branches on the right side, and that accidental posterior straying of the excision does not lead to involvement of the major portion of the artery before its curve backwards into the posterior parasagittal zone.

Having defined the site and depth of the top of the tumour by careful brain needling, the first step should be a linear incision in the dura from the parasagittal area to the subfrontal zone laterally. When the intracranial tension is appreciably raised, this incision should then be deepened with division of cortical arteries and veins, working initially about 2 cm parasagittally to avoid the major anterior cerebral circulation until the top of the tumour is reached. The superior aspect of the tumour capsule frequently contains very large tumour veins, and it is best to avoid disturbance of these at this stage. The capsule of the tumour is then followed laterally until the roof of the orbit is reached, and medially to reach the falx. Provided the falx is approached with care, and the level of the excision has been correctly planned, the stretched branches of the anterior cerebral artery passing along the top of the tumour at this stage will be only fronto-polar branches and may be divided with confidence. If the approach is made to these vessels from lateral to medial as described, then their distribution and anatomy may enable the surgeon to realise before it is too late that he has carried the planned frontal excision too far posteriorly and has involved himself with the major anterior cerebral trunk, when of course these vessels must be meticulously preserved. This decision having been made, the polar frontal lobectomy may be completed and parasagittal and falcine venous attachments clipped and coagulated. Such a polar excision will usually serve to control even quite considerably

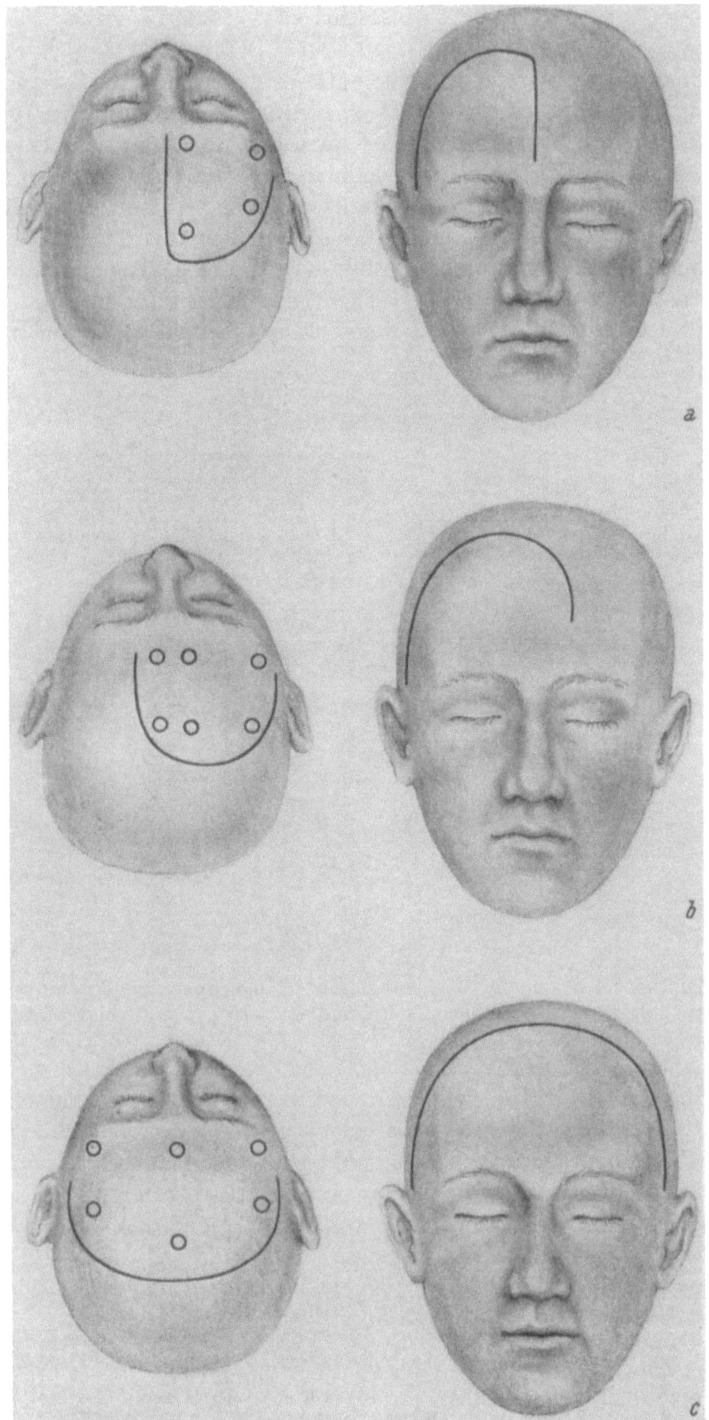

Fig. 9. Various incisions used for the approach to subfrontal and jugum sphenoidale meningiomas

raised intracranial pressure and, in the author's experience, the use of mannitol is now seldom required. The position achieved is now shown in Fig. 10. It is at this stage wise and convenient to pursue dissection a little way backwards along the top of the capsule of the tumour, defining the extent and degree of adhesion, particularly of the anterior cerebral branches. Where these are closely applied to the capsule they should not be further dissected at this stage. In moderate-sized tumours, however, it may be possible even thus early to determine that the adhesion to anterior cerebral vessels is slight, and also by passing laterally along the roof of the orbit to define the outer end of the sphenoidal wing and, thereafter

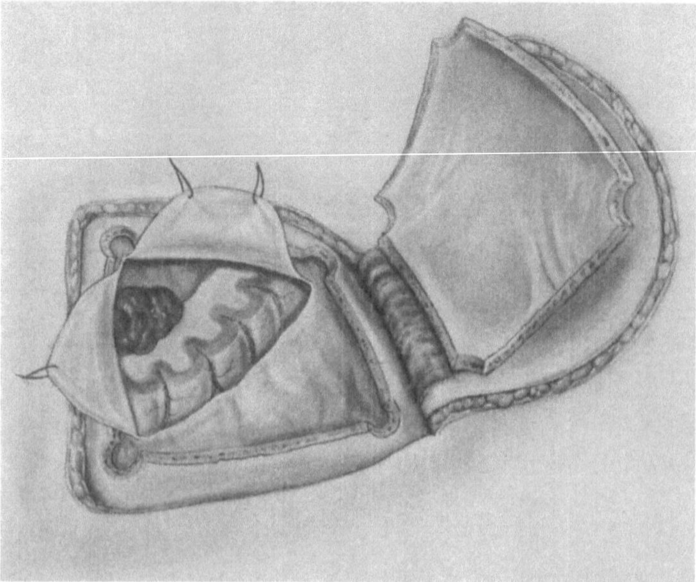

Fig. 10. Excision of a subfrontal meningioma. Dural opening and the preliminary polar frontal lobectomy have been completed, exposing the surface of the tumour

passing medially, with gentle retraction of the preserved portion of frontal lobe to define the position of the right optic nerve even thus early. The clue to the position of the optic nerve is the olfactory tract, which may be picked up round the top of the tumour capsule and followed back to the point where it crosses the sphenoidal wing. Dissection towards the sphenoidal wing may at the same time enable release of CSF from the lateral aspect of the chiasmal cistern by gentle breach of the arachnoid lateral to the optic nerve and carotid artery. In large masses, however, it is generally impossible to consider such extensions of the exposure at this stage.

Removal of the Centre of the Mass

The next step in an average-sized or large mass should therefore be the coagulation of a portion of the capsule and the commencement of exenteration of the mass. Here attention should be drawn to the angiographically displayed arterial supply from the ethmoidal vessels. The method of exenteration of the centre of the tumour will be determined by the tumour's consistency. Rarely will be possible suction coagulation on a small metal sucker or exenteration of the centre of the mass with a large sucker. More commonly, the typical fibrous, stringy meningioma septa will demand that the tumour be gutted with diathermy loops, and in hard and fibrous masses this is the only method available (Fig. 11).

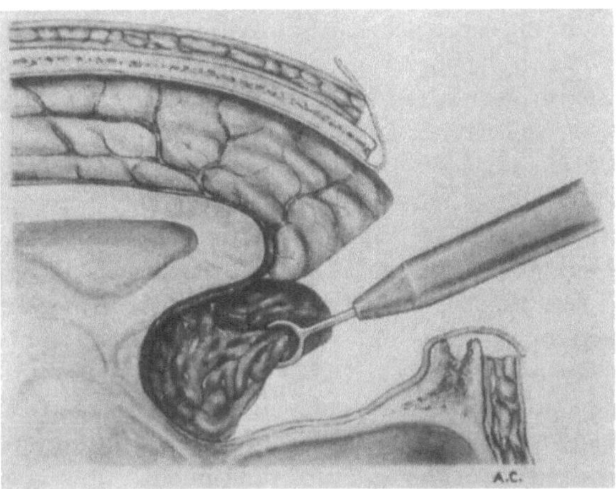

Fig. 11. Excision of a subfrontal meningioma. The loop excision towards the base and the entering blood supply is shown, dissection now being pursued upwards towards the anterior cerebral circulation

The Entering Blood Supply

Under these circumstances, loop excision should be carried down to the bone of the olfactory groove where the entrant vessels may be coagulated, and the aim should be gradual backward sloping extension of the approach on the olfactory groove until the major vasculature has been coagulated. Particularly with a large arterial input from the ethmoidal vasculature, this process may require coagulation of the entrant vascular branches after each cut with the loop; it may involve considerable blood loss and the expenditure of a good deal of time. The use of a large sucker to evacuate the field, with an available small metal sucker to coagulate the bleeding points, may appreciably lighten this task. When the bleeding from the subfrontal area has been adequately controlled, and only then, the dissection of the attachment of the capsule of the tumour from the subfrontal brain may begin.

Definition of the Anterior Cerebral Circulation

At this point loop excision upwards, under the capsule, will thin the capsule sufficiently to enable it gently to be depressed from the brain, and the vascular attachments to be outlined. A frequent major difficulty at this stage is the large, capsular veins of the tumour which often run forwards and medially to the falx, or backwards and laterally to enter venous tributaries of the spheno-parietal sinus associated with the middle cerebral veins. As the top of the capsule is detached from the brain so, with release in local tension provided by the exenteration of the centre of the mass it is possible, by drawing the capsule gently down, to define the extent of adhesion of the anterior cerebral vessels to the top of the mass. Rarely, it may be necessary to divide the attachment of the vessels to the top of the mass with sharp dissection, and under these circumstances the use of magnification is advisable. In general terms, however, a very large subfrontal tumour presents problems of management which demand an expeditious approach, and magnification during the rapid central exenteration of a mass, particularly in the face of considerable haemorrhage, is neither useful nor advisable. Where both anterior cerebral vessels are involved, and where the mass is very large, access to the top of the leftsided portion of the tumour may be improved by division of the falx from below upwards to the lower border of the sagittal sinus. Should further access prove necessary, then a bone flap across the midline will have been used, in which case the anterior portion of the sagittal sinus and polar frontal veins on the left side may be divided at this stage, and gentle lateral retraction of the left frontal lobe used to enable the dissection of subfrontal branches of the anterior cerebral on the left side from the top of the capsule. It cannot be over-emphasised, however, that adequate exenteration of the centre of the mass should precede such capsular dissection, as the facility of capsular dissection is much enhanced by the capacity to retract the capsule down into the cavity created by excision of the centre of the tumour.

The anterior cerebral circulation having been defined, it is usually found that the major anterior cerebral vessels lie in fairly thick arachnoid and separate from the dome of the tumour postero-superiorly. If this should not prove to be the case, then the potential extension of the tumour onto the sphenoidal wing should be suspected, since actual involvement of the terminal carotid artery and the proximal anterior cerebral artery in the pure olfactory groove or suprasellar tumour is rare.

The Dissection of Optic Nerves and Chiasm

After the vascular dissection has been pursued to a stage in which the major vessels have been freed from the top of the tumour, dissection in the right parasellar area should be undertaken. The key to the approach here is the line of the sphenoidal wing, which may be picked up lateral to the edge of the tumour and pursued medially to define the position of the right optic nerve. In olfactory groove tumours, this is usually overlaid by the posterior extension of the mass and is not directly involved in its attachment. The right postero-lateral corner of the tumour may now be dissected and the line of the right optic nerve used as a guide to join the two regions of dissection in the superior and postero-lateral aspects of the capsule. As a rule, it is best to pursue the right optic nerve round the mass until the direction and line of set of the chiasm are apparent, by which time the anterior cerebral circulation will have been entirely freed from the top of the capsule and the capsule may then be directed downwards, forwards and to the right, away from the left postero-superior angle of the mass. At the same time the line of the planum sphenoidale will have been revealed, and the capsule may be folded gently away from the left side of the optic apparatus. In very large tumours, it may be necessary at this stage to approach the left side of the lesion through the left half of the bifrontal approach indicated in such conditions, and to pick up the left optic nerve separately by definition of the inner end of the sphenoidal wing on the left side. In the author's experience this is rarely necessary but, where the surgeon has little experience of the handling of such tumours, it is a valuable adjunct in the exposure.

It is regrettably true that even with apparent preservation of olfaction before operation, the excision of a bifrontal olfactory groove meningioma is invariably accompanied by total destruction of the sense of smell.

Handling the Ethmoidal Vascular Supply and the Hyperostosis

As a rule, the region of the hyperostosis in the olfactory groove will contain the major ethmoidal feeding branches. During the excision of the centre of the mass, it is wise to leave sufficient soft tissue on the bone to enable coagulation and arrest of haemorrhage. When the tumour has been excised, however, the management of the hyperostosis and its contained vessels must be considered. Usually suction coagulation with the metal sucker will remove the bulk of tumour, and a large hyperostosis may be trimmed with bone forceps. The recurrence rate of such lesions, however, is so low that heavy diathermy coagulation of the attachment is usually sufficient to prevent recurrence, and over-zealous treatment of the hyperostosis may well result in perforation of the top of the ethmoidal air sinuses, especially if they are "blistered" into the base of the hyperostosis. Provided this is recognised by the surgeon and repair of the frontal fossa with fascia lata or pericranium promptly undertaken no harm will ensue but, if heavy coagulation of the floor of the fossa perhaps with pursuit of a bleeding vessel by coagulation in its foramen with the blunt hook is undertaken (a useful trick), then CSF rhinorrhoea may result unless the area is covered with pericranium even in the absence of apparent perforation.

The Technique of Excision of Meningiomas of the Jugum Sphenoidale

The major added problem presented by meningiomas of the jugum or more posteriorly attached lesions on the planum, and perhaps even more by the true meningiomas of the suprasellar area, is their much greater involvement with the chiasmal apparatus.

As a corollary and in compensation, however, the sheer bulk of meningiomas of the jugum sphenoidale is less than those of the olfactory groove, implicit in their earlier involvement of the chiasmal apparatus bringing the patient to surgery at an earlier stage in the growth of the mass.

In the author's experience, a unilateral frontal flap is invariably adequate for approach to a true suprasellar tumour. Extensive bifrontal retraction in posteriorly placed subfrontal lesions is undesirable, leads to damaging psychological sequelae and to total loss of olfactory sensation, which may be avoided if dissection is pursued entirely from the right side.

Control of ICP

In meningiomas of the planum or jugum sphenoidale, wedge excision of the frontal pole is seldom indicated unless the mass is very large, in which case it attains the characteristics of a posteriorly placed lesion in the olfactory groove. The usual, more posterior placement, of the mass means that no uncapping of the tumour is possible through a lobectomy of permissible extent, and the control of intracranial pressure in very large tumours of the jugum area is therefore much more difficult. Fortunately, brain needle tapping of the ventricle may reduce the tension sufficiently for formal dural opening, and an early approach to the lateral aspect of the chiasmal cistern in the right parasellar area may ensure drainage of CSF and further slackening of brain tension. If, however, intracranial pressure appears high and is not controlled by ventricular tapping, then mannitol should be given before the dura is opened. In the author's experience, this is virtually never necessary. The dural opening in such cases should be through a curved subfrontal incision extending from the midline to the lateral angle of the orbit, with a re-entrant incision extending backwards to the outer end of the sphenoidal wing (Fig. 12).

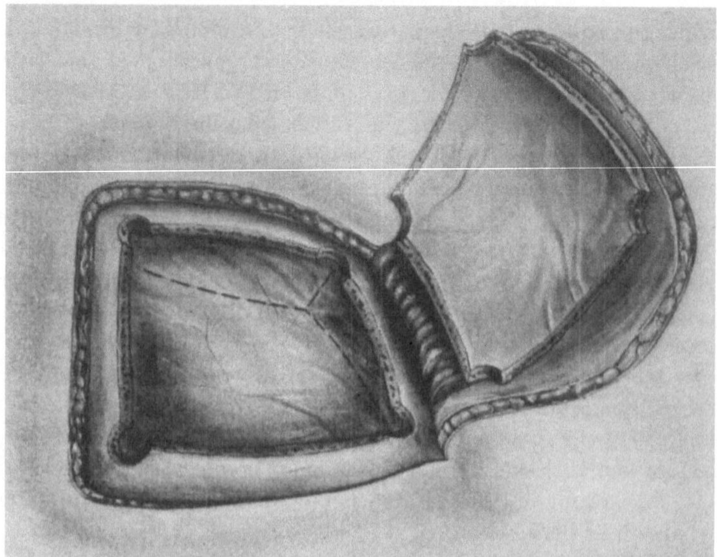

Fig. 12. Dural incision for approach to a meningioma of the jugum sphenoidale

Preliminary Orientation

Gentle elevation of the frontal lobe from the orbital plate is then commenced, the olfactory tract defined and divided on the right side at this stage, and dissection pursued backwards along the olfactory groove and planum sphenoidale until the anterior border of the meningioma is reached. This dissection should be carried back in the midline so that the premature encounter with an ill-defined right optic nerve is avoided. Depending upon the size of the mass, it may now be possible to pass round the right side of the attachment of the mass to pick up the medial end of the Sylvian fissure on the right. Opening the arachnoid carefully over the Sylvian fissure will enable drainage of CSF, and may enable the surgeon at this stage to pick up the terminal carotid artery and the right optic nerve. Not uncommonly, however, the involvement of the optic nerve by the tumour is so complex that definition cannot be achieved thus early, and dissection should therefore continue on the presenting face of the tumour until an adequate area has been cleared to enable the tumour to be entered. In this regard must be mentioned the occasional unusual behaviour of anterior clinoidal tumours, one of which in the author's series, presenting as an apparent jugum mass, extended between the internal carotid artery and optic nerve in such a way that the optic nerve was carried medially by the expansion of the mass, and lay just above the jugum on the lower aspect of the capsule of the tumour. In dissection of the capsule of a tumour well offset from the midline, arising from the area of one anterior clinoid, this rare medial displacement of the ipsilateral optic nerve must be borne in mind before coagulation of the capsule and dissection towards the jugum, lest the optic nerve be damaged at an early stage before its unusual displacement is recognised.

Gutting the Tumour

This caution observed, the capsule should be coagulated, a portion of it excised close to the bone of the planum, and dissection within the tumour itself pursued to diminish the bulk of the centre of the mass. Once again, the key is to continue close to the bone of the planum, coagulating the entrant vessels as they pass through the jugum or planum so that the subsequent dissection of the dome of the capsule is rendered virtually bloodless. Care is necessary as dissection proceeds posteriorly along the planum so that one does not pass over the curve of the jugum prematurely into the suprasellar area. The avoidance of damage to the chiasmal apparatus in the excision of these masses demands that rocking of the tumour in the embrace of the chiasmal apparatus be avoided. When dissection too far posteriorly within the mass itself is pursued before the chiasmal apparatus is defined, at least in part, then such physical disturbances of the optic apparatus are impossible to avoid.

Identification of the Chiasmal Anatomy

Having dissected, therefore, on the jugum as far back as the entrance of the major blood supply, the line of dissection should now be turned to separation of the capsule from the gyrus rectus and from encircling branches of the anterior cerebral arteries. Extensive adhesion to the gyrus rectus is not uncommon, but excision of brain in this area is not recommended until some idea of the line of displacement of the chiasmal structures has been obtained. It is therefore essential, at an early stage, having freed sufficient of the top of the capsule to enable it to be gently pulled down and inwards towards the left and forwards from the right parasellar area, that a search be made for the right optic nerve and the right carotid artery. Here, dissection under the operating microscope and bipolar coagulation may be invaluable. A very stretched optic nerve may be difficult to delineate from the capsule of the tumour, and inspection under the operating microscope will greatly enhance this differentiation. If the operating microscope is used, it will be important to place suitable self-retaining retractors, and the author's preference has been for the Yasargil double-bladed self-retaining retractor, fixed to a base plate on the skull. External fixation through the appropriate fitment to the operating table itself may be preferred.

The involvement of the right optic nerve may either be by tumour overlying it, or by tumour passing down the posterior face of the jugum sphenoidale into the suprasellar area and displacing the nerve laterally so that the line of the nerve is almost antero-posterior. True encirclement of the optic nerves is rare, but not uncommonly the tumour overlaps the optic nerve from above and extends also beneath the optic nerve between the nerve and the carotid artery in a dumb-bell expansion in the parasellar zone. This represents a particularly dangerous involvement of the nerve, since only its lateral aspect is immediately visible and since it is very difficult to determine in which direction the nerve is running. Occasionally, of course, attachment to the anterior clinoid extends much further lateral and the problem therefore becomes not that of a suprasellar meningioma but of a mixed suprasellar and inner third sphenoidal wing tumour. Regrettably, while the suprasellar meningioma is almost invariably capable of total excision, the inner third sphenoidal ridge meningioma is not so amenable to surgery. A decision may therefore have to be made that, if the optic apparatus is completely encircled by an inner third sphenoidal attachment of the mass, involvement of the carotid artery is likely and that a portion of the tumour may have to be left behind. Assuming, however, a true suprasellar or jugum mass, definition of the right optic nerve and carotid artery will enable gradual pursuit of the dissection along the dome of the tumour from the right side. At this point it must be admitted that, where the suprasellar extent of the mass is large, the bulk of the tumour above and behind the optic apparatus on the right side may effectively prevent dissection of the capsule downwards and inwards into the cavity of the centre of the tumour from the right side at this stage. Having defined the anterior limit of the right optic nerve and the right side of the chiasm, therefore, it is wise to pursue dissection into the left side of the capsule with gentle elevation of the left subfrontal zone and gradual exenteration of the left side of the mass on the jugum and anterior clinoid, until the point of crossing of the olfactory tract and the sphenoidal wing indicates the probable level of the left optic nerve. It is, fortunately, rare that both optic nerves are encircled or appreciably embarrassed by the tumour; these masses almost invariably involve one nerve much more than the other and, if heavy involvement of the right makes dissection on the right impossible, it will usually be found that the left is rather freer and, having been identified, dissection may be pursued in the left parasellar zone to separate the left side of the chiasmal apparatus from the tumour. From the right-sided approach, postero-superior extensions on the left are very much easier to reach and evacuate centrally than those on the right, where the surgeon is working round a corner as it were, and it may therefore be possible at this stage, even with a very posteriorly placed extension, to define the medial aspect of the left optic nerve, the left carotid and the left half of the chiasm, and to exenterate the bulk of the mass from left to right in its posterior aspect.

A further point to note here is that the displacement of the chiasmal apparatus, in the author's experience, is frequently skew so that, while one optic nerve is held fairly well forwards with the tumour bulging to some extent behind it, the other tends to be flattened by the mass from above and in front. The chiasm frequently occupies a very oblique line as a result. When, therefore, the right optic nerve is found to be held at its foramen and the mass clearly extends substantially in the parasellar area behind and to the right, the left optic nerve will usually be found to be overlaid by the mass and the chiasm, to pursue a highly oblique course from right anterior to left posterior. Less commonly, and rather more easily, the tumour may overlie the optic apparatus completely so that the chiasm is pressed downwards and backwards behind the mass. Some indication of this latter deformity will have been given by AEG. It is in the handling of dumb-bell extensions of the mass above and behind the chiasm into the anterior third ventricle that most difficulty will be experienced, and here the best line of approach, having defined both optic nerves and the anterior chiasm, is to pursue dissection down through the centre of the mass onto the top of the diaphragma sellae. By this means, in the true jugum mass or one in which the attachment does not extend completely back along the diaphragma sellae, it may be possible to pass into free subarachnoid space below the posterior extension of the tumour and thus to define the posterior extent of the capsule. This may then be thinned down by gentle suction coagulation, thus enabling the whole mass to be gently drawn down from the region of the third ventricle.

Fortunately, the free knob of tumour extending into the chiasmal and prepontine cistern is seldom so hard as to require loop excision, but it may nevertheless present formidable difficulties in dissection, which are exacerbated the more posteriorly the attachment on the diaphragma sellae extends. Where such a posterior extension is accompanied by extension along the medial end of the sphenoidal wing with encirclement of terminal carotid or proximal anterior cerebral arteries on one or other side, the problems of excision reach their maximum. Even here, however, unless the terminal carotid artery itself is encircled, it may be possible under the operating microscope to dissect the proximal anterior cerebral artery free of the mass. Division of the proximal anterior cerebral artery, even in the presence of angiographically demonstrated adequate filling from the opposite side, is not recommended, as it almost invariably risks sacrifice of key perforating vessels from the anterior cerebral to the anterior part of the internal capsule, and has been responsible for the author's only fatality in 40 cases. Even a grossly attenuated anterior cerebral, regrettably, often fulfils an important function. It is probably better, if freeing of the mass from tight anterior cerebral attachment proves impossible, to leave that portion of the tumour attached to the anterior cerebral and remove the remainder of the mass as far as possible.

Division of one optic nerve, even when that is functionless on pre-operative assessment, is generally of little help in the excision of meningiomas in this region. If the tumour so involves the region of the carotid artery and the optic foramen as to render its dissection under the operating microscope impossible, then division of the optic nerve alone is unlikely appreciably to enhance the prospects of removal, and the tumour should probably be considered unsuitable for total excision. Under the operating microscope or direct vision, the forward extension of a little knob of tumour into the optic foramen on the medial side or beneath the optic nerve may be detectable. Preliminary plain films will have indicated the probability that the optic foramen is itself involved, but usually this small knob of tumour may be picked cleanly from the foramen by dissection with a blunt hook.

The Treatment of the Dural Attachment

The dural attachment of these masses is usually to the hyperostosis in the region of the jugum, if that is present. This may be substantially offset towards one anterior clinoid or another, and may extend down across the posterior face

Table 1

Total cases		40 (16 male, 24 female)				
Age range		23–74 years				
Age distribution	21–30	31–40	41–50	51–60	61–70	71 +
	1	2	17	12	7	1

Approx. site of origin

Olfactory groove (S) only	Mixed olfactory grooves and jugum	Jugum and anterior clinoids only	Jugum and suprasellar area	Involvement of inner third sphenoidal wing and vessels in jugum and clinoidal tumour
5	13	11	7	4*

Incomplete removal	3	all in this group*
Operative deaths	1	all in this group*
Operative mortality	2.5%	
Involvement of visual function	33	
Improvement in visual function post-operatively	26	

* Two cases who presented with complete blindness, one in one eye and the other in both eyes, showed no significant recovery of vision, vision in the completely blind case recovering to perception of light in one eye at the end of a month. Useful vision was, however, recovered in several optic nerves whose visual acuity had been reduced to counting fingers pre-operatively.

of the jugum into the true suprasellar area. In the author's experience, heavy coagulation of the dura and the hyperostosis has been sufficient to prevent recurrence. Here again, however, where large vascular channels traverse the bone, it may be wise to cover the heavily coagulated base of the tumour with pericranium or fascia lata lest CSF rhinorrhoea develops in the post-operative phase. During coagulation of the base of the tumour, of course, care must be taken not to involve the optic foramina, but the classical suprasellar mass confines its attachment to the superior and posterior faces of the jugum and does not usually involve the circumference of the optic canals themselves.

Closure

In the closure of unilateral frontal excisions for olfactory groove or jugum lesions, where the procedure has begun with an excision of the medial part of the frontal lobe, and the dural incision has involved a small triangular flap based medially, this flap should be carefully repaired with interrupted black silk sutures. If the frontal sinus has been opened, the defect may be plugged with a piece of temporal muscle, in turn covered by a small piece of pericranium. The pericranium may be held in place by sutures or by the application of spots of tissue glue such as Histoacryl Blau. Where the defect is flat, a piece of lyophilised dura cut to size and held in place with Histoacryl Blau, is also effective. The bone flap is replaced and held in place with a single perforating stitch through its centre tied over a silver clip, and anchored by multiple pericranial sutures of black silk. The temporal muscle is carefully closed anteriorly to avoid an unsightly defect, and the anterior burrhole filled with bone dust collected during the opening. The scalp is then repaired with a layer of interrupted black silk sutures in the pericranium tied so that their knots are deeply placed, and a single layer of skin stitches in black silk. A suction drain left in the subgaleal space prevents the collection of blood beneath the flap in the first few days. It should be removed after 48 hours, at which time the skin stitches may also be removed.

Closure of Bifrontal Craniotomy for Large Orbito-Frontal Meningiomas

Particularly where the frontal sinuses are large, the bifrontal flap very frequently opens the frontal sinuses fairly extensively. In addition, with a very large bilateral subfrontal mass, a large cavity may be left, the falx is divided and the dura may be very difficult to repair accurately. It is the author's practice in such circumstances to leave the bone flap out, the flap itself being stored in a solution of saline containing antibiotic (Penicillin and Streptomycin), and kept at a temperature of — 4 °C under sterile conditions until it may be replaced in some three months' time. Any defect in the frontal sinuses is occluded with temporal muscle, covered with pericranium or lyophilised dura, and the scalp closed in two layers without drainage. Aspiration of the scalp flap may well be necessary for a few days to combat the local collection of CSF and, where the subfrontal cavity is very large, it may be necessary in addition to supplement post-operative management by episodic lumbar punctures if proteinous excretion from the cavity gives rise to a phase of transient impairment of CSF absorption. The bone flap may be replaced without difficulty after some months when the intracranial pressure has completely settled, and disturbance of the frontal sinus closure can be readily avoided at this time.

References

Cushing, H., Eisenhardt, L., **1938**: Meningiomas: Their Classification, Regional Behaviour, Life History and Surgical End Results. Springfield/Ill.: Ch. C Thomas.

Ehlers, N., Malmros, R., **1973**: The suprasellar meningioma. Acta ophthalmol., Copenhagen, Suppl. *121*.

Fusek, I., Kunc, Z., **1969**: Causes of unsuccessful surgical treatment of suprasellar meningiomas. Cesk. Neurol. *32*, 279—283.

Guillaumat, L., **1937**: Les méningiomes supra-sellaires. Thèse, Paris.

Olivecrona, H., **1967**: The surgical treatment of intracranial tumours. In: Handbuch der Neurochirurgie, Bd. IV/4. Hrsg. H. Olivecrona, W. Tönnis. Berlin-Heidelberg-New York: Springer.

Zülch, K. J., **1956**: Biologie und Pathologie der Hirngeschwülste. In: Handbuch der Neurochirurgie, Bd. III. Hrsg. H. Olivecrona, W. Tönnis. Berlin-Göttingen-Heidelberg: Springer.

Microsurgical Approach to Acoustic Neurinomas

M. G. Yaşargil, R. D. Smith, and J. C. Gasser

Neurosurgical Clinic, University of Zurich (Switzerland)

With 17 Figures

Contents

I. Introduction

The diagnostic and surgical problems of tumors of the cerebellopontine angle have fascinated neurologists, neurosurgeons, otologists and neuroradiologists for decades as evidenced by the great outpouring of papers and monographs on this subject. Of the tumors in this area, the acoustic neurinoma has a special significance in two respects;

1. It is the commonest tumor found in this area (65–70%).

2. The origin of the tumor is in the inner ear, an area generally considered in the speciality province of the otologists. It grows from here into the cerebellopontine angle, thereby coming into the speciality area of the neurosurgeons. It is no wonder that development of surgical technique should have interested both the otologist and the neurosurgeon.

At the outset of this discussion it should be noted that the paper will be confined to the neurosurgical aspects. In addition the development and the results of classical neurosurgery will not be summarized, since this has already been masterfully done in the publications of Cushing (1917), Dandy (1941), Olivecrona (1940, 1967), McKenzie and Alexander (1955), Pool and Pava (1957), Drake (1967), and Pertuiset *et al.* (1970). It would furthermore be unfair to compare the results of classical neurosurgery with those of microneurosurgery, since the incomparably better working conditions of today were not at the disposal of the pioneering generation of neurosurgeons. It must however be noted here that the achievements of microneurosurgery are fundamentally based on the keen perceptions and hard won experience of this earlier generation.

II. Microtechnique

As long as 50 years ago, otologists employed the operating microscope and microinstruments for operations in the area of the middle ear. The use of the operating microscope for translabyrinthine exploration (House 1961), for subtemporal transpetrosal exploration (Kurze and Doyle 1962) and for suboccipital transmeatal exploration (Rand and Kurze 1965) captured the imagninations of modern neurosurgeons and neurootologists. Since that time advances in the field of microneurosurgery have been concentrated on extirpation of tumors in the posterior fossa as well as in microvascular and aneurysm surgery. There have been introduced new microscopes, microinstruments, bipolar coagulation technique, electric high speed drill, a nerve stimulator, self-retaining brain retractors, and microsuture material for vessel and nerve operations. The knowledgeable employment of these materials demands a basic course of experience in the laboratory, with use of instruments in fine dissection, preparation and suturing techniques of vessels and nerves, experience with bipolar coagulation, and skilful handling of electric drilling instruments.

One special problem has been the difficulty of changing the position of the operating microscope during operation. A mobile microscope has now been developed wherein the balanced microscope head with its accessories (photo-, film- and television cameras) can be moved weightlessly in horizontal and vertical directions with a mouth switch. The hands of the surgeon remain free to carry out the necessary maneuvers of the operation undisturbed (Figs. 1a–c). Especially important in operations in the posterior fossa is that the microscope head has a substantial range of motion such that it can be rotated through an arc of about 250°.

Stable immobilization of the head is obtained with the patient in the sitting position by use of three-point skeletal fixation (Mayfield-Kees) (Figs. 2a–c).

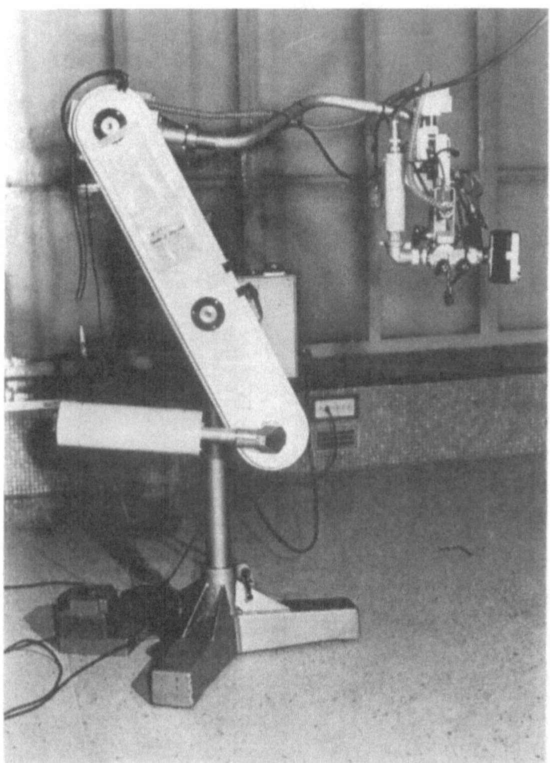

Fig. 1a. Balanced mobile microscope with electromagnetic brakes

Another pressing problem in neurosurgery demanded a solution, *i.e.* the unstable retraction of a brain spatula held by an assistant. To guarantee the precise, stable, and at the same time gentle retraction necessary, a flexible retractor arm of adjustable tension which could be fixed extracranially was developed. A heavy angulated metal rod is secured to a side rung of the operating table with a hand torqued bolt. A sterile metal head with several insertion sites for retractors is fitted over the other end of this rod. One or more retractors arms can then be placed in various positions to allow maximum flexibility in direction of retraction (Figs. 3a–b). This system also allows the craniotomy to remain small as will be described below (Fig. 8).

III. Surgical Anatomy of the Cerebellopontine Angle

A thorough knowledge of the anatomy of the cerebellopontine angle gained from several excellent textbooks is indispensible to the neurosurgeon. This is

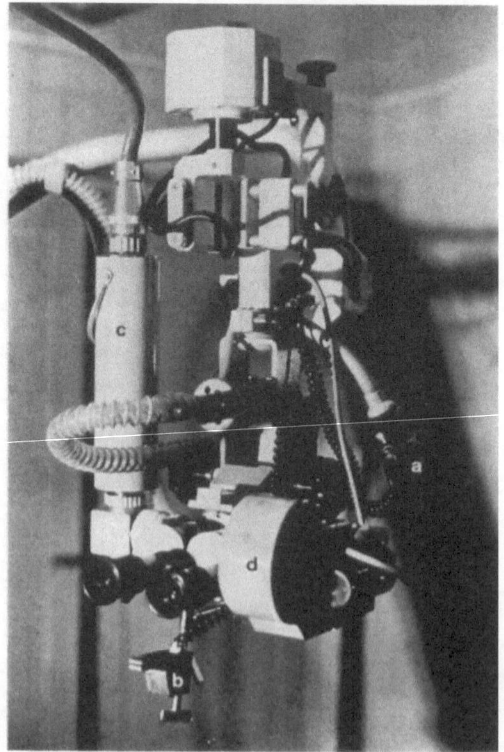

Fig. 1b. Close-up of microscope head: *a* handswitch, *b* mouthswitch, *c* closed circuit television camera, *d* movie camera

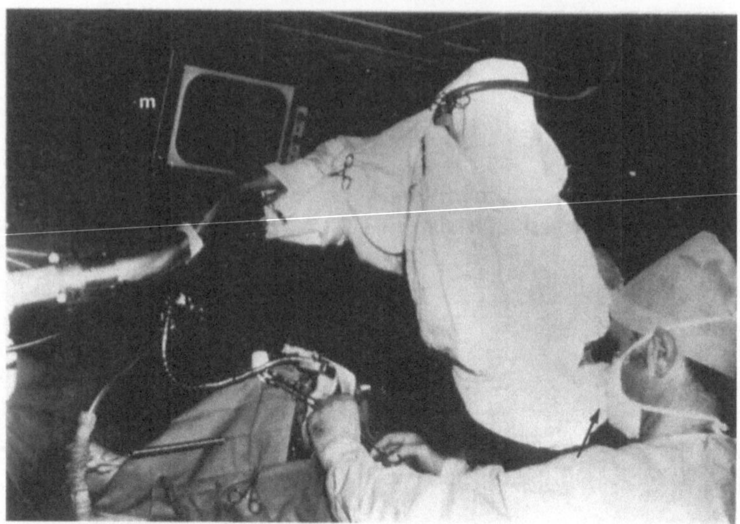

Fig. 1c. Sterile draped microscope in position. *m* television monitor. Black arrow points to mouthpiece

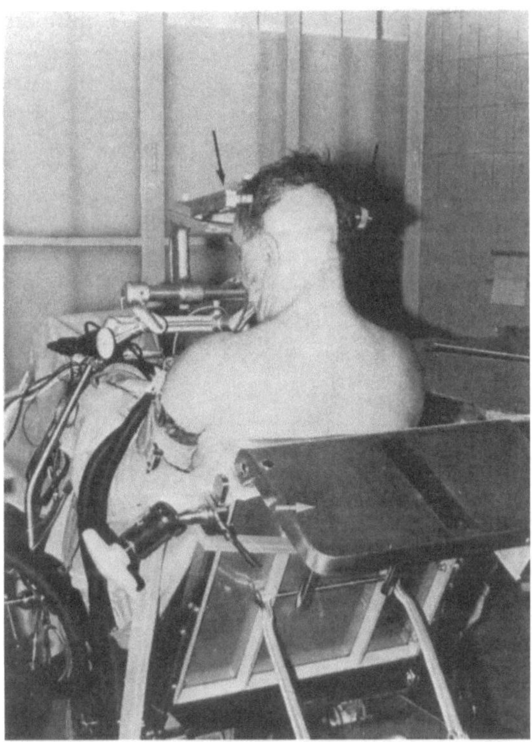

Fig. 2a. Position of patient for left sided cerebellopontine angle exploration. Posterior view. Black arrows indicate position of three point skeletal fixation device. White arrow points to the adjustable surgeon's arm rest

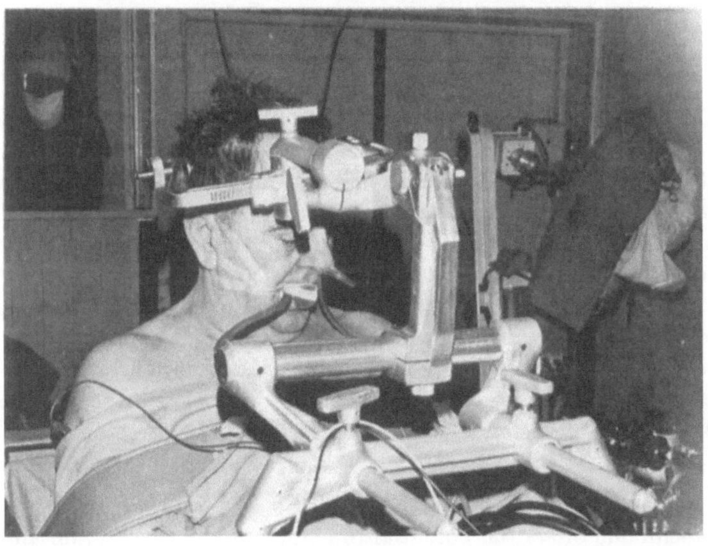

Fig. 2b. Frontal view of patient in skeletal fixation device. Arrow points to microscope draped and ready for use

however not sufficient; the surgeon must work in a different anatomical perspective, and must be familiar with the variations of structures caused by the mass and growth patterns of tumors. Details of various anatomical structures seen radiologically including by computerized tomography (changes in the petrous bone, position of the nerves, pons and cerebellum and position and varia-

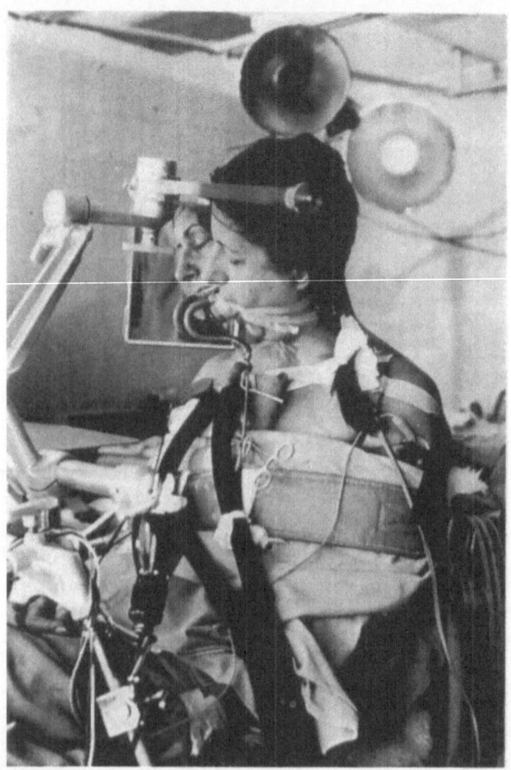

Fig. 2c. Use of mirror with patient positioned for right sided exploration

tions of the blood vessels, and finally the size and exact position of the tumor) provide of course very important information. One is dealing however with a two dimensional representation. Even with the availability of stereoscopic roentgenograms, the surgeon must abstract the desired information and transpose it into three dimensional space. Following this the surgeon must recognize the magnified structures in a funnelshaped craniotomy, and be able to operate with the impression that he is not outside the area of exploration but rather standing in the center of field. Microtechnique therefore demands a special level of anatomical knowledge of the cerebellopontine angle.

1. Subarachnoid Cisterns

Microtechnique offers the potential to carry out the exploration and extirpation of a tumor within the subarachnoid space and to protect the arteries, veins and nerves lying in various subarachnoid cisterns. Resection of the cerebellar

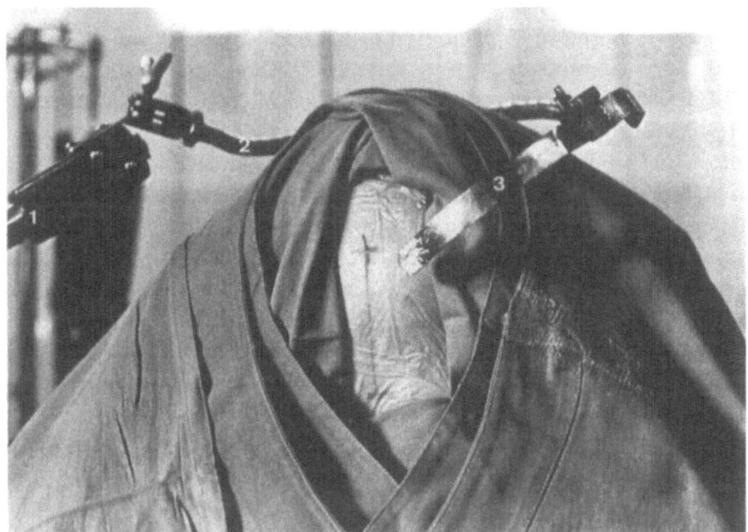

Fig. 3a. Extracranially fixed self-retaining retractor in position for left sided exploration. *1* Coupling head, *2* retractor arm is adjustable to position and tension, *3* malleable spatula blade

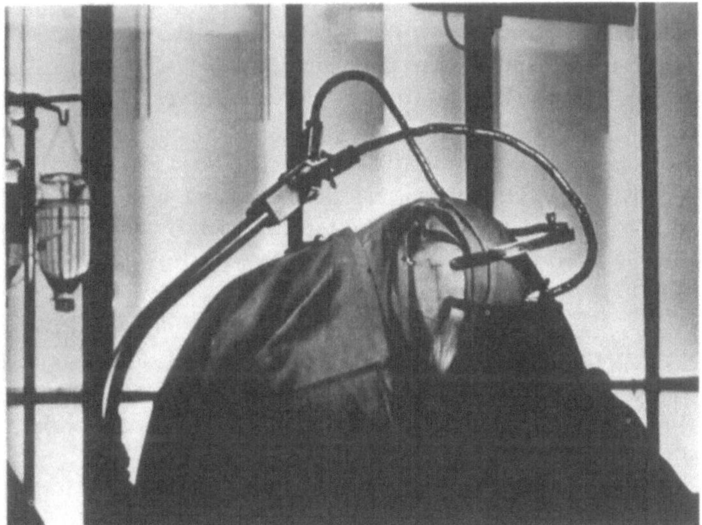

Fig. 3b. Two retractors in position

hemisphere is contraindicated, even with large tumors of the cerebellopontine angle, because the cisterns infiltrated with blood will no longer be clearly demarcated and the exploration of the tumor, the nerves and the vessels cannot be carried out under proper visualization. This limitation of space demands a precise knowledge of the structure and interrelationships of the basal cisterns. In this small area many subarachnoid cisterns come together and the anatomy of these cisterns and their relationship to the fourth ventricle through the foramen of Luschka have therefore a special importance for neurosurgeons. The following papers can be recommended: Key-Retzius (1875), Liliequist (1959), Epstein (1966), DiChiro (1967), Leighton (1971), McClure-Wilson (1972) and Samii (1974). These very carefully performed studies on cadaver material and observations of cisternograms answer primarily the needs of the neuroradiologist. Giving full recognition to the excellent work referred to above, it must be noted that many structures are destroyed by fixation and section. With radiological studies, including stereoscopic roentgenograms, numerous details will not be adequately portrayed and very fine partitions go unrecognized. Microsurgical technique has permitted these subarachnoid cisterns, demonstrated through meticulous effort by the above named authors, to be observed *in vivo* and studied in minute detail. The small area of the cerebellopontine angle is not occupied by a single cistern, the cerebellopontine cistern, but includes also the lateral cerebellomedullary cistern and the prepontine cistern. At the caudal border of these is the premedullary cistern, craniodorsally the superior cerebellar cistern, the quadrigeminal cistern, and ambient cistern and finally cranioventrally the interpeduncular cistern. These cisterns can vary as regards their size, extent, structure and borders. The entrance and exit points of the nerves and arteries are frequently strengthened with thickened, multiple arachnoid fibers. The foramen of Luschka opens at times into the cerebellopontine cistern, at times into the lateral cerebellomedullary cistern and occasionally into the prepontine cistern.

Fig. 4 provides a general view of the cisterns in the cerebellopontine angle including which nerves and arteries they contain.

The cisterns contain the following arteries and nerves:

a) Cerebellopontine Cistern

Nn. V, VII, and VIII, anterior inferior cerebellar artery, auditory artery, branches of the petrosal vein and the brachium pontis vein, the interbrachial vein, vein of the lateral recess and the transverse pontine vein.

b) Lateral Cerebellomedullary Cistern

Nn. IX, X, XI, and XII, vertebral artery and the first segment of the posterior inferior cerebellar artery to the undersurface of the cerebellar tonsil where it enters the posterior cerebellomedullary cistern, the vein of the lateral recess, the medial tonsillar vein and the lateral medullary vein.

c) Prepontine Cistern

N. VI, the basilar artery to the upper edge of the pons where it enters the interpeduncular cistern, the origin of the anterior inferior cerebellar artery and the transverse pontine vein.

d) Quadrigeminal Cistern

N. IV, the superior cerebellar artery, precentral cerebellar vein, end of the basal vein of Rosenthal, lateral mesencephalic vein and the posterior mesencephalic vein.

e) Ambient Cistern

Lateral to the quadrigeminal cistern just at the edge of the tentorium a part of this cistern is still visible where the trochlear nerve curves forward and the superior cerebellar artery turns backward to run in the quadrigeminal cistern.

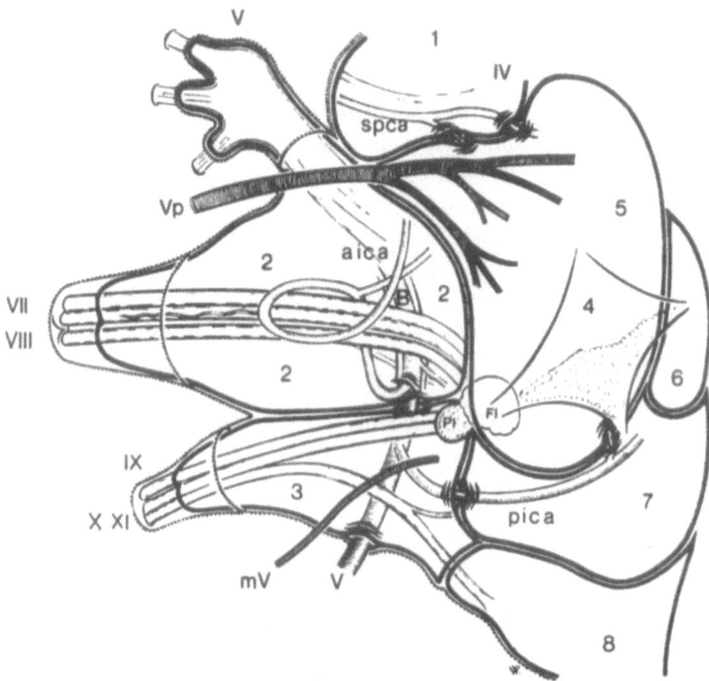

Fig. 4. Diagram of cerebellopontine angle to demonstrate cisternal relationships. *1* Ambient cistern, *2* cerebellopontine cistern, *3* lateral cerebellomedullary cistern, *4* fourth ventricle, *5* superior cerebellar cistern, *6* cerebellar hemisphere, *7* cisterna magna, *8* cervical subarachnoid space, *spca:* superior cerebellar artery, *aica:* anterior inferior cerebellar artery, *pica:* posterior inferior cerebellar artery, *B* basilar artery, *V* vertebral artery, *Vp* petrosal vein, *mV* medullary vein, *Fl* flocculus over the foramen of Luschka, *Pl* choroid plexus. The cranial nerves are designated by Roman numerals

The basal vein of Rosenthal lies in this cistern and proceeds for a short segment into the quadrigeminal cistern where it joins the great vein of Galen.

The petrosal vein courses in the upper edge of the superior cerebellar cistern and on the lower edge of the quadrigeminal cistern where the tributaries of the marginal veins, the lateral pontomesencephalic vein and the veins in the cerebellopontine cistern, the vein of the lateral recess, the brachial vein and the interbrachial pontine vein, join it.

The cisterns accompany the cranial nerves out of the intracranial cavity into the jugular foramen, internal auditory meatus and Meckel's cave. The variability of extension of the subarachnoid space into the area of the inner ear has been impressively demonstrated by pantopaque cisternography (Fisch and Weber 1972, and Portmann *et al.* 1973).

2. Relationship of the Tumor to the Cistern

The acoustic neurinoma takes its origin from the intracanalicular segment of the vestibular nerve, or very infrequently, the cochlear nerve, so that the origin of the tumor is in fact outside the subarachnoid space (epiarachnoidal or extra-arachnoidal). With medial growth of the tumor, the wall of the cerebellopontine cistern is pushed medially until there is a duplication of these layers of arachnoid or even a triplication as the boundaries of the lateral cerebellomedullary, prepontine, and quadrigeminal cisterns are reached (Figs. 5a–c).

By inadequately defining the plane of dissection, one runs the risk of dissecting between the arachnoid and tumor capsule on one hand or between the arachnoid and the pia on the other, gaining the impression that the tumor has invaded these boundaries and has extended into the brain substance, which rarely if ever occurs. It must be appreciated that even a nodular, irregular tumor indenting the surface of the pons and cerebellar hemisphere until they are virtually unrecognizable nevertheless actually stops within the arachnoid. An exact knowledge of the subarachnoid space, its contents and its boundaries, is of the greatest importance in the extirpation of these tumors.

IV. Operative Technique

Successful exploration of the cerebellopontine angle depends on several factors such as the position of the patients, the incision, the extent of the craniotomy and whether it should include resection of the arch of the atlas, and finally a specific technique of exploration and resection of the tumor.

Four methods have been advocated in approaching acoustic neurinomas:

1. Subtemporal transpetrosal exploration (tumors 2–6 mm).
2. Subtemporal or suboccipital transtentorial exploration.
3. Translabyrinthine exploration (tumors 10–25 mm).
4. Suboccipital transmeatal exploration.

The diagnosis of very small acoustic neurinomas has been infrequently made so that only the cases of House (1961), Kurze and Doyle (1962), and Fisch (1968)· have been published in which the subtemporal transpetrosal route was used in exploration and extirpation. In these cases the function of not only the facial nerve but also the cochlear nerve could be saved.

The subtemporal or suboccipital transtentorial exploration of medium and large tumors which was first described by Fay (1931) and later advocated by Rosomoff (1971) and Morrison and King (1973) has the hypothetical advantage that the facial and cochlear nerves can be visualized directly on the surface of the tumor. The method has the disadvantages of retraction on the temporal and occipital lobes, sacrifice of the temporal and occipital basal veins, venous stasis, and collection of blood and cerebrospinal fluid in the basal cisterns such as to obscure the important arteries and nerves on the back of the tumor.

On the advice of Panse (1904), several surgeons successfully approached acoustic neurinomas by the translabyrinthine route in the early part of the century—Kümmel (1909), Quix (1911), Schmiegelow (1915) and Zange (1915). House (1961) resurrected this method 50 years later with the use of the operating microscope, high speed electric drill and microinstruments and worked out the microanatomy of this region. His achievements stimulated neurosurgeons to consider similar techniques. The translabyrinthine is the approach most commonly used by otolaryngologists today. However the question is not yet answered whether

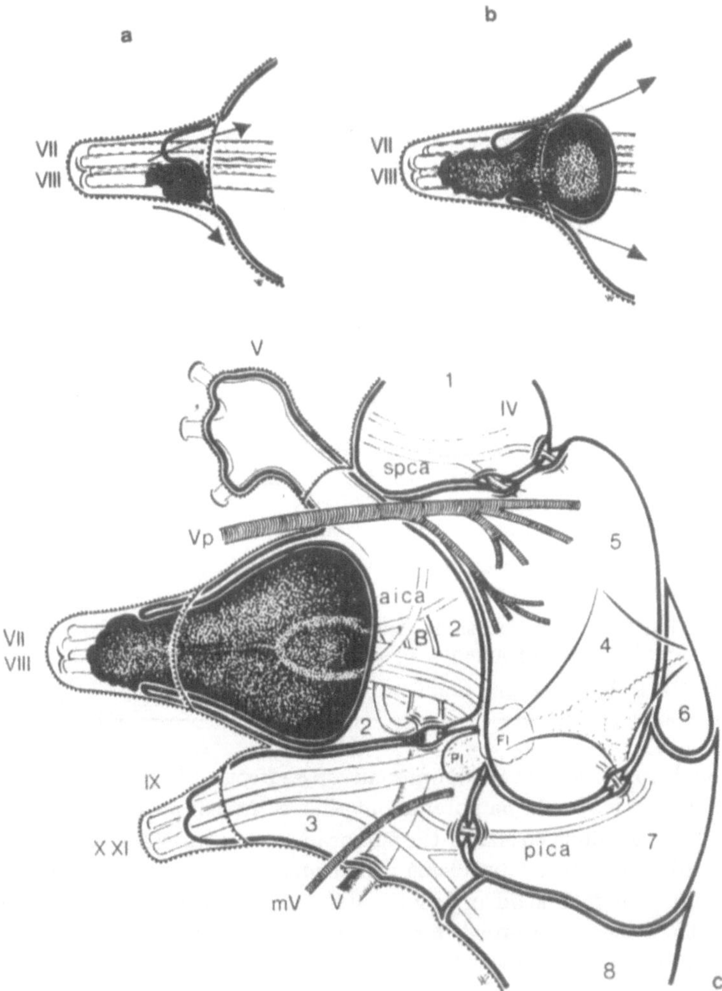

Figs. 5a, b, and c. Represent growth of an acoustic neurinoma from the internal auditory meatus into the cerebellopontine angle. Numbers and letters same as Fig. 4

translabyrinthine exploration is an appropriate procedure for extirpation of an acoustic neurinoma. In the majority of cases, large tumors cannot be completely removed through a translabyrinthine approach. Even in so-called medium-size tumors, important vessels remain hidden from the surgeon approaching the tumor laterally. From the first House appreciated these difficulties and introduced a combined approach—a translabyrinthine exploration followed by a suboccipital approach—in close association with a neurosurgeon [Hitselberger and Raney (1964), Hitselberger and House 1966]. The advantage of the translabyrinthine approach, exposure of the meatal portion of the tumor and freeing of cranial nerves VII and VIII in this area in preparation for a second operation, must be weighed against certain disadvantages—not only the second course of anesthesia and wound healing for the patient, but also the loss of clear planes in the subarachnoid space from blood and adhesion following the first procedure. It can be seen from Table 1 that most of the tumors were larger.

Table 1. *Tumor Size and Preoperative Condition of Patients* (September 1967 until July 20, 1976)

	Grade				Number of patients
	I	II	III	IV	
< 2 cm	4	—	—	—	4
2–3 cm	15	12	3	—	30
3–5 cm	3	33	26	7	69
5 < cm	2	18	29	19	68
	24	63	58	26	171

Grade I Patients with only vestibulocochlear symptoms.

Grade II Patients with vestibulocochlear symptoms and a weak or absent corneal reflex.

Grade III Patients with additional symptoms of cerebellar and lower brain stem dysfunction (dysphagia, dysarthria, ataxia, papilledema).

Grade IV Bedridden patients unable to care for themselves.

Although tumor size has a definite adverse effect on the patients preoperative status (Table 1), it should be pointed out that technical problems for the surgeon are not related as much to size of the tumor as to its consistency and relationships to surrounding structures, problems which must be solved at the time of operation. Tumors may be solid or gelatinous and have a thin or a well-developed capsule. They may be fibrous, fatty or perhaps have a soft center but be exceedingly tough peripherally. In addition to the parenchyma, the vascularity of the tumor is a factor that cannot be adequately evaluated preoperatively. A further important factor is the degree of adherence of the capsule to arteries, brainstem and especially with cranial nerves VII and VIII. A relatively small or medium-size tumor can be exceedingly adherent to these nerves while a large tumor may displace and elongate the nerves with only minimal adherence. Special difficulties are encountered in the removal of the fibrous acoustic neurinomas from young patients with neurofibromatosis. These tumors are fibrous, bleed readily and can be densely adherent to the surrounding nerves. One must also consider the seldom encountered cystic tumor which following evacuation of the cyst presents no problem in removal. More often however these cystic tumors fill the entire subarachnoid space, extending into every conceivable crevice of the basal structures and have dense adhesions to the vessels and nerves. With the use of the microsurgical technique and a clear strategy, all tumors can be removed through a standard size craniotomy with minimal damage to vital structures. How this is accomplished will be presented in the following paragraphs.

1. Position on the Operating Table

The first patients done in this series were placed in the prone position. This position was unsatisfactory because marked venous oozing obscured the operative field making operative manipulations hazardous. The lateral decubitus

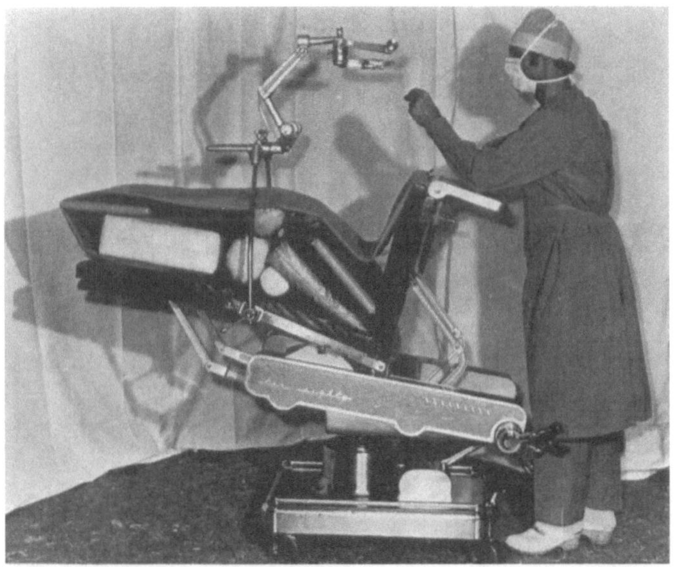

Fig. 6. Operating table with skull fixation apparatus and adjustable arm rest

position is advocated by otologists as being more favorable for the translabyrinthine approach. This approach is utilized also by some neurosurgeons who fear the risk of air embolism in the sitting position. In general however neurosurgeons in the last 10 to 15 years have found the sitting position described by De Martel (1931) as most acceptable. Blood and cerebrospinal fluid flow naturally out of the wound leaving the operative field bloodless and clearly visible. The sitting position has been used in all patients in this series since 1968 as well as for other posterior fossa operations, occipital craniotomies and cervical laminectomies. In 280 cases during this period there was not one symptomatic case of air embolism. With the anesthesiologist using increased intrathoracic pressure and intermittent compression of the jugular veins, it is possible to visualize small venous bleeding points in soft tissue and bone and control them with coagulation or wax. An armrest attached to the operating table combat fatigue from long periods of standing (Fig. 6).

2. Positioning the Patient

The patient is seated in the upright position on several layers of cushions to allow variation in height on the operating table. The legs are wrapped with elastic bandages and elevated about 20 degrees above horizontal.

The head is held in the three point skeletal fixation device designed by Mayfield and Kees slightly flexed forward (one should be able to place a hand between the chin and the manubrium to guard against compression of the trachea and jugular veins). The head is turned about 30 degrees toward the side of the tumor so that the retroauricular area with the slightly arched mastoid process comes to lie in the middle of the operating field (Fig. 7). In this way, a direct entrance to the cerebellopontine angle parallel to the pons will be gained.

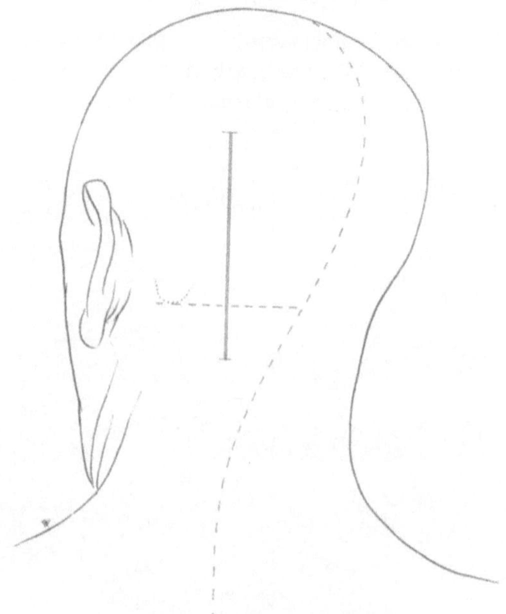

Fig. 7. Skin incision

3. Incision and Craniotomy

A paramedian retroauricular retromastoid incision of about 6–7 cm is made and the skin undermined about one cm on each side. Galea and periosteum in the occipital and suboccipital area including over the mastoid process are elevated and retracted. The origin of the splenium capitis muscle is lifted from the skull and retracted with clamps, but the deeper muscles are not disturbed. It is not necessary to divide the muscles below the horizontal ridge at the base of the occipital bone.

The first burr hole is placed at the level of the external occipital protuberance, three fingerbreadths lateral to it, just above the transverse sinus. The second burr hole is placed over the mastoid and the third 3 cm medial to it over the suboccipital area. The two sides of this triangle of bone are sawed through, and with a high speed electric drill the base is grooved with a slight curve such that a bone flap 4 cm long and 3 cm wide can be removed. The mastoid air cells are drilled down until the sigmoid sinus is visible. The use of a high speed electric drill has the advantage that the emissary veins in the mastoid bone can be followed and coagulated just before their entrance into the sigmoid sinus.

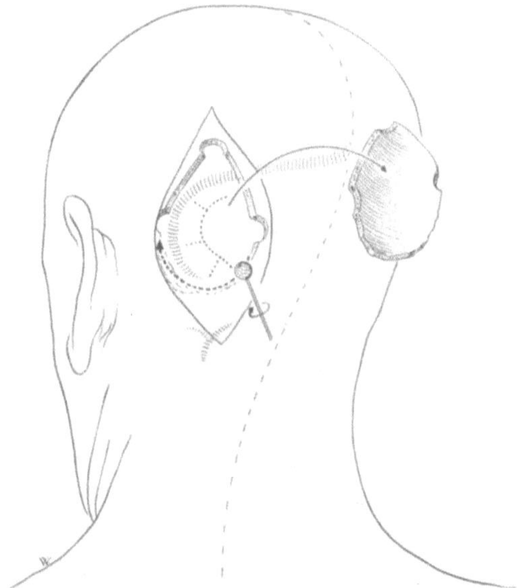

Fig. 8. Bone flap

With removal of the mastoid air cells laterally and basally at least 30 degrees increased angle of vision into the cerebellopontine angle will be gained, so that the surgeon can later move the operating microscope to inspect the entire area from the tentorial edge to the foramen magnum and can perform any necessary maneuvers in these areas. The primary goal of the surgeon should not be to resect cerebellar tissue or employ excessive retraction, but rather to be aggressive in removal of mastoid bone to create the necessary operating space. The opened air cells are packed with muscle and bone wax. The arch of the atlas is not removed. It is also unnecessary to extend the craniotomy medially in the direction of the foramen magnum. Enlargement of the craniotomy over the cerebellar hemisphere may mislead the surgeon into excessive retraction of this rather soft tissue. The surgeon must accustom himself to operating through a small opening in a funnel-like space and to identify and handle structures under these conditions (Fig. 8).

4. Opening of the Dura

When the dura is especially tense the surgeon should not feel compelled to extend the craniotomy mediobasally or to remove the arch of the atlas but should instead use this trick: A one centimeter incision is made in the dura one centimeter medial to the sigmoid sinus and just above the basal occipital line. A second incision mediobasally creates a small triangle based inferiorly (Figs. 9a–b). The laterobasal corner of the cerebellar hemisphere is retracted about 5 mm upward and medially to expose the lateral cerebellomedullary cistern. This cistern is opened above or below the spinal accessory nerve releasing cerebrospinal fluid. The danger of tonsillar herniation by sudden pressure alterations with a large tumor already associated with increased intracranial

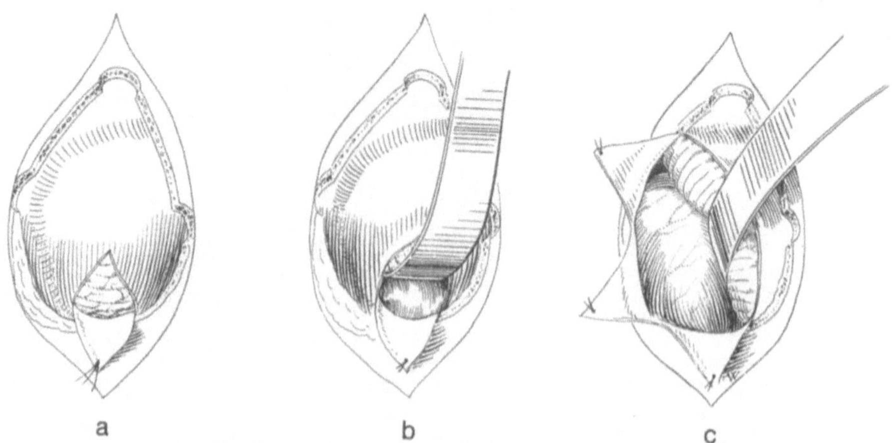

Fig. 9a. Triangular dural flap in laterobasal area
Fig. 9b. Exposure of lateral cerebellomedullary cistern
Fig. 9c. Dural incision after opening of lateral cerebellomedullary cistern

pressure is now obviated, since the cisterns over the foramen magnum and tonsil will have been decompressed by this maneuver. From this point the dura will be opened in a standard way. A 2 cm semicircular incision of the dura is made approximately 1½ cm from the transverse and sigmoid sinuses. The dura lateral to this incision is opened as three triangles with the sinuses forming their bases and these sections of dura are retracted with sutures over the sinuses (Fig. 9c). Should a sinus inadvertently be opened, a small hole can usually be closed with microsuture material or microclips. If during the craniotomy a larger opening is made in the sinus, a beaten muscle stamp is applied to the rent and fixed with a bonding agent, Aron alpha (Aron Alpha A®, Sankyo Co., Ltd., Japan), so that the lumen of the sinus remains open.

In opening the lateral cerebellomedullary cistern, one must pay special attention to a small vein which originates in the lateral area of the biventer lobule of the cerebellum, collects fine branches from the tonsil and medulla and courses laterally and caudally crossing the cistern and spinal accessory nerve to enter the dura in the area of the jugular foramen.

After the release of cerebrospinal fluid, the cerebellar hemisphere will spontaneously recede cephalad. The dura is not opened over the lateral cerebellar hemisphere, but is left untouched. A quadrangular flat cottonoid strip is laid over the dura and the ventrolateral cerebellar hemisphere and the hemisphere retracted 1 to $1\frac{1}{2}$ cm medially. The retractor blade is held by a self-retaining retraction arm fixed extracranially as described above.

5. *Evaluation of the Tumor*

With retraction of the cerebellar hemisphere, the dorsolateral surface of the tumor will now be visible, not infrequently covered with a cystic appearing collection of yellowish cerebrospinal fluid, loculated in the partially obstructed cerebellopontine cistern. After evacuation of this yellow fluid, fine arterioles and venules will be seen to lie between and bridge the tumor capsule and the retromeatal dura. These must be completely coagulated so that they do not rupture and fill the subarachnoid space with blood, obscuring the operative field from the beginning of the operation. It is important that the duplication of arachnoid over the tumor be meticulously opened in an entirely blood free field and that the subarachnoid cisterns on the medial wall of the tumor remain uninjured during further dissection. It is not necessary to determine the entire extent of the tumor initially either for the purpose of determining its size or the position of the important arteries. This would demand excessive retraction on the cerebellar hemisphere and cause pressure on the brainstem.

After coagulation of the dural surface and vessels in the retromeatal area the question still remains of whether it is more advantageous to begin removal in the meatus in order to identify the facial and vestibuloacoustic nerves and from here proceed medially, or to first free the tumor from the brainstem to protect it from retraction and pressure. Whether initial dissection medial or laterally is advocated, it is important to first gut the tumor in order to gain working room.

The arachnoid membranes over the dorsal surface of the tumor are divided and separated to expose the tumor capsule. A six to eight millimeter area of the tumor capsule is coagulated and a circular incision made (Fig. 10a). Through this small opening it will be possible to remove much of the tumor tissue with the aid of sharp dissectors, rongeurs and if the tissue is soft with a sucker. The opening in the tumor capsule should not be too large, because in vascular tumors blood will be lost into the subarachnoid space obscuring adequate visualization of the structures. Should bleeding from a large artery or vein inside the tumor ensue, this can be grasped and coagulated. Should diffuse parenchymatous oozing occur, it is recommended that pressure with muscle, Gelfoam, Spongostan or Tabotamp be used. With progressive hollowing out of the tumor center, increased space will be gained and the peripheral parts of the tumor can be drawn toward the center (Fig. 10b). This maneuver dispenses with the need for any further retraction than that established at the beginning of the dissection. The stable position of the retractor blade on the lateral edge of the cerebellar hemisphere prevents mechanical injury.

6. *Mobilization of the Tumor* (Fig. 11)

After the center of the tumor has been evacuated, the arachnoid duplication between tumor capsule and the cerebellopontine and cerebellomedullary cisterns

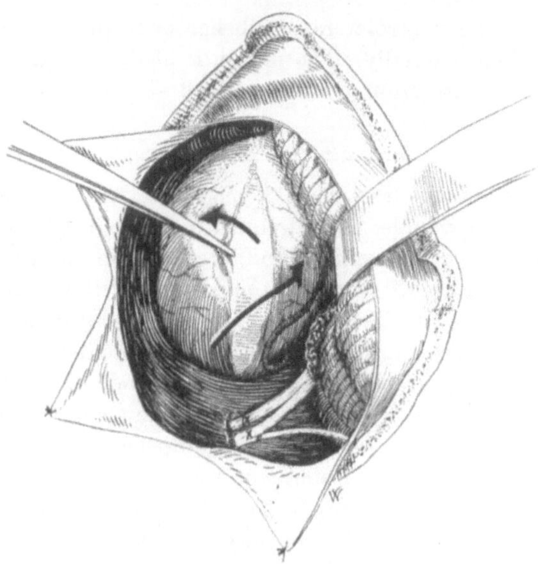

Fig. 10a. Opening of arachnoid membranes over tumor capsule. Roman numerals denote cranial nerves

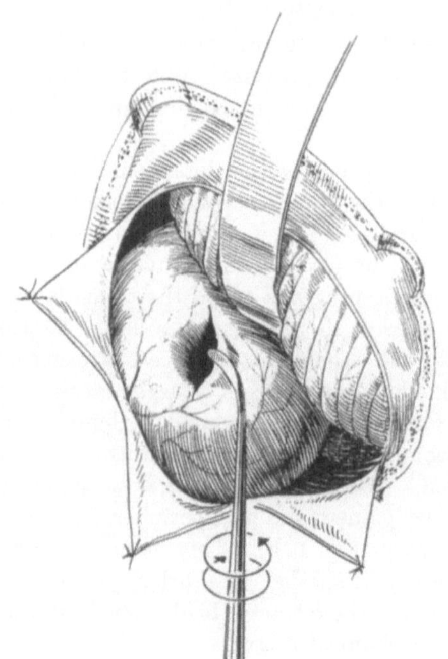

Fig. 10b. Internal decompression of tumor

is opened and the branches of the anterior inferior cerebellar artery to the tumor coagulated. The glossopharyngeal and vagus nerves are mobilized from the tumor capsule and care taken to free a loop of the anterior or posterior inferior cerebellar artery should either be encountered here. The use of a flat sponge to push these structures medially is recommended. In this phase of the operation it is the aim of the surgeon to advance along the supraolivary fossa to indentify the foramen of Luschka at its upper point. Here are found the converging point of the above named cisterns as well as the junction of the

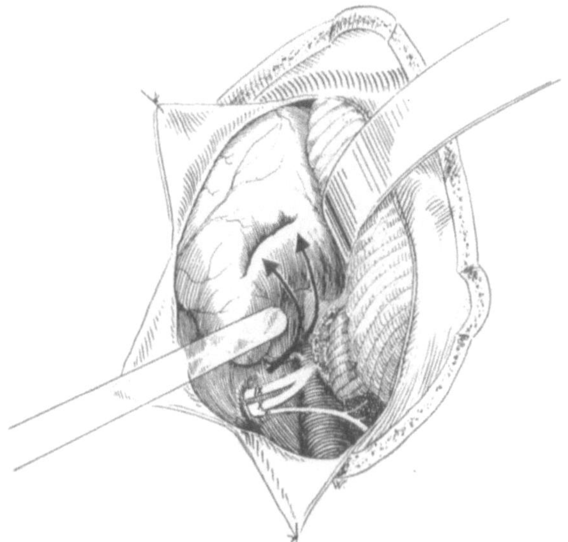

Fig. 11. Retraction of tumor from supraolivary fossa. Roman numerals denote cranial nerves

vertebral artery with the basilar artery, the origin of the anterior inferior cerebellar artery and posterior inferior cerebellar artery coursing through. Here are also found the beginning layers of arachnoid which form the cisterns, the lateral exit of the tela choroidea and the superficial membrane of the lateral recess of the fourth ventricle. The choroid plexus protrudes from the foramen of Luschka and comes to lie beneath the flocculus. The supraolivary fossa is divided in its mid portion by the pontomedullary sulcus. Beneath the sulcus cranial nerves IX and X exit from the medulla and diverge caudally and laterally, while nerves VII and VIII enter above the sulcus from a lateral cranial position near the pons. Above these lies the vein of the lateral recess.

With protection of the arachnoid membranes and the above mentioned vessels and nerves in this area, the tumor must be mobilized and retracted laterally avoiding injury to the pia of the medulla, pons and laterobasal portions of the cerebellar hemisphere. The freeing of this corner allows recognition of the position and course of the major vessels, above all the anterior and posterior inferior cerebellar arteries and their branches. In order to explore this corner, cranial nerves IX and X are followed along the cerebellomedullary cistern from the caudal pole of the tumor medially to their origin. The flocculus and choroid plexus are dissected free and the tumor gently retracted laterally from above. At an angle of 90° above the pontomedullary sulcus, the pontine origins of cranial nerves VII and VIII are visualized at the foot of the flocculus as 1 ½–2 mm thick white bands. In most cases these nerves have been displaced 1 ½–2 cm by the ventromedial section of the tumor. Even in tumors which deeply indent the pons and flatten the pontomedullary sulcus, these nerves may be dissected free as far as the origin of the trigeminal nerve at the top of the brachium pontis (Fig. 12). As long as it is possible to remain in the subarachnoid space, leaving

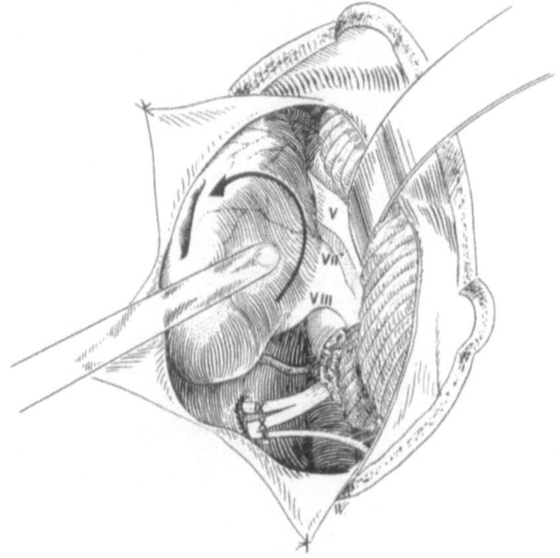

Fig. 12. Retraction of tumor from pons. Roman numerals denote cranial nerves. The anterior inferior cerebellar artery is seen coursing laterally from the vertebro-basilar trunk. The choroid plexus and flocculus overlie cranial nerves IX and X

a layer of arachnoid on the tumor and a layer on the pons, even where the tumor has extended deep into the pons, successful extirpation can be achieved without injury to the pia mater, or pontine veins and arterioles. Should one stray across this anatomic boundary, the desired cleavage of the tumor from the brainstem will not be attained. The arachnoid covering the pons will be torn, the tumor veins and junctions of the pontine veins will be injured and possibly small arterioles from the anterior inferior cerebellar and basilar arteries will be disrupted. In such a case, one has the impression that the tumor has become intimately adherent to the pons and to the blood vessels. To avoid such a potentially catastrophic state of affairs the arachnoid membranes must be given special close attention.

Cranial nerves VII and VIII becomes splayed out on the ventromedial section of the tumor and often on the ventral surface of the tumor become nothing more than a transparent membrane on the tumor capsule. These splayed fascicles may course over the cranial pole of the tumor. On occasion the facial nerve will be elongated cranially and come to lie above the upper edge of the trigeminal nerve before looping caudally to run to the porus acousticus. It is advisable not to attempt further dissection of these nerves beyond that point where they begin to become widened and thinned, but rather to leave them temporarily and concentrate on mobilization of either the antero-inferior area, the postero-superior area or the antero-superior portions of the tumor. The transition of the vertebral artery into the basilar artery and the cranially directed abducens nerve are found. These structures have little adherence to the tumor capsule and a precise dissection is obtained. (In 8 cases it was observed that the origin of the abducens nerve was split into two parts by the anterior inferior cerebellar artery.)

Over the cranial pole of the tumor it is necessary to protect the trigeminal nerve and the petrosal vein and its branches, there are usually no significant adhesions. The trigeminal nerve however is very sensitive to mechanical stimulation which may result in a sudden elevation of blood pressure. It is therefore advisable to proceed very cautiously in this area and to dab the nerve with 1% procaine during dissection. In especially large tumors, parts of the tumor can extend cranially into the quadrigeminal, ambient, crural and interpeduncular cisterns thereby requiring isolation of the trochlear nerve (34 cases), oculomotor nerve (2 cases), superior cerebellar artery, pontomescenphalic vein or the basal vein from the tumor capsule. After mobilization of the caudal, medial and cranial parts of the tumor from the brain stem, additional tissue can be removed from the tumor center and the just mobilized portion of tumor pressed centrally with cottonoid patties. Gutting of the tumor should not be vigorously undertaken with an attempt to evacuate the entire content initially because the danger exists that the tumor capsule will suddenly be penetrated allowing blood to ooze along the ventral tumor surface blocking the basal cisterns. In addition by tearing the tumor capsule the facial nerve may be injured. The repeated intermittent coring of the tumor with continuous gentle pulling of the mobilized medial part of tumor toward the center, allow the surgeon to assess the extent and thickness of the remaining tumor tissue and thus proceed with further tumor removal. The freed nerves and vessels are covered with thin rubber strips cut from sterile surgeons gloves and in this way protected from damage during further instrument manipulation. After at least half of the tumor along the brainstem has been dealt with by the above described hollowing out, mobilization and piecemeal removal, the surgeon can turn his attention to the lateral part of the tumor.

7. *Exploration of the Meatal Portion of the Tumor*

The internal auditory meatus is on the average 12 mm long and 5–15 mm wide depending on the size of the intrameatal extension of the tumor. Dorsally, the bone is generally quite compact and is 10–15 mm thick. The dura invaginates the meatus as it turns up onto the porus acousticus such that in drilling away bone from the porus, the contents of the meatus are protected by a sheath of dura. In drilling the bone it is important that initially a shallow wide area 10 to 12 mm be created rather than a small deep groove (Fig. 13). A cutting steel burr is used initially. Deeper into the bone progressively smaller diamond drills are employed. For left sided tumors the electric drill should turn in a clockwise direction and for right sided tumors in the opposite direction. One must pay special attention not to remove too much bone in the direction of the jugular foramen, since occasionally an outpouching of the jugular bulb extends to this area and can be injured. Drilling too far laterally on the petrous bone will endanger the facial nerve in the Fallopian canal. In those cases where the patient still has useful hearing and the cochlear nerve may be saved, it is important to preserve the cochlea and the superior semicircular by not drilling more than a few millimeters lateral to the porus acousticus.

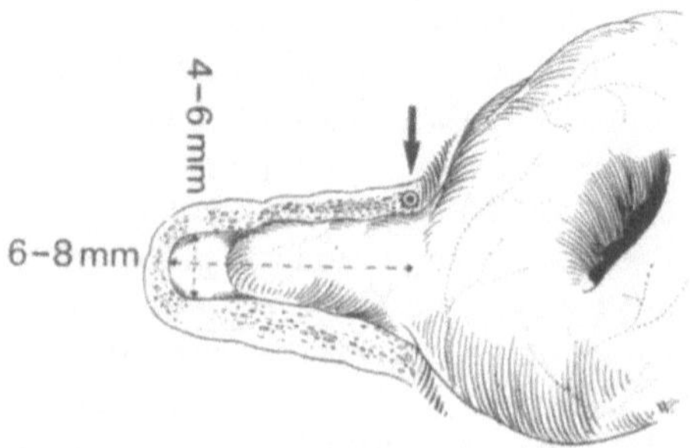

Fig. 13. Intrameatal portion of tumor. Arrow points to usual position of large artery in petrosal bone encountered when opening internal auditory meatus

Within the meatus there are few if any significant adhesions between the tumor and nerves, such that this tongue of tumor can be stripped back to the porus acousticus without special difficulty. With the magnification provided by the operating microscope, the nerves are recognized as white bands although they can sometimes become very flattened and almost transparent. The facial nerve is always found on the superior cranial wall of the meatus although in 3 cases the nerve had turned dorsally in the meatus and come to lie on the dorsal surface of the tumor (Fig. 14). In exiting from the porus into the intracranial cavity, the nerve will suddenly angle 60 to 80° from its horizontal course and splayed and flattened will come to lie on the ventral surface of the tumor. Here dense adhesions between the tumor capsule, arachnoid and dura must be divided with attention payed to dural arteries from the vertebral and middle meningeal arteries as well as arteries coming from the petrous temporal bone (see Fig. 13). It is recommended that the dura be somewhat elevated from the bone and bone wax pressed into osseous bleeding sites. At times a loop of the anterior inferior cerebellar artery will have a short segment within the dura in the area of the porus. It is not advisable to attempt to dissect the artery from this dura but better to cut out the piece of dura and leave it attached to the artery.

Perhaps the most difficult part is the ventrolateral portion, 1–1½ cm long and wide where the tumor capsule and the nerves are routinely extremely adherent seeming to have almost grown together. In 11 cases, even with the greatest degree of magnification available on the operating microscope it was no longer possible to distinguish between tumor capsule and nerve tissue. To

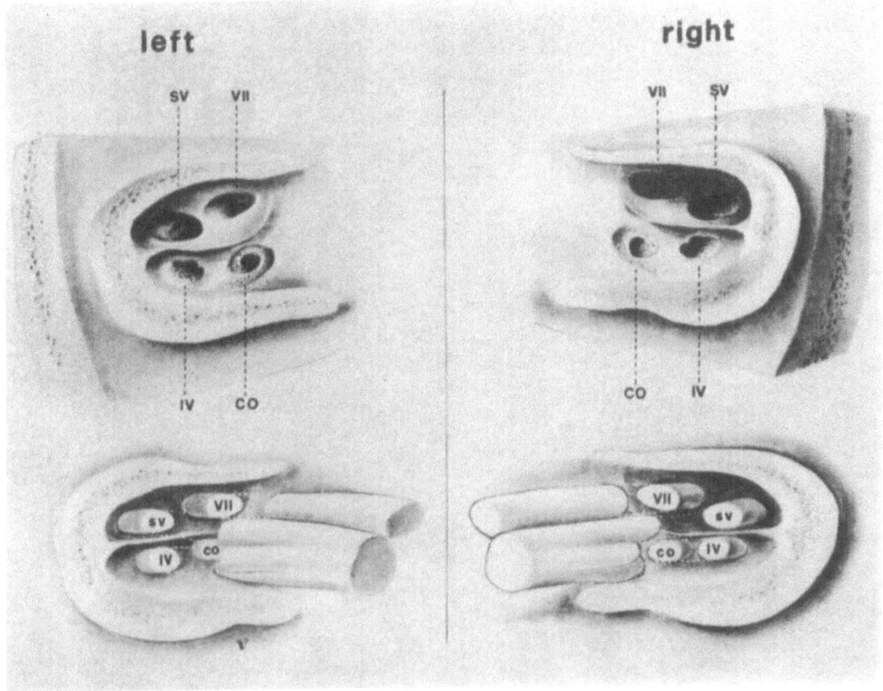

Fig. 14. Anatomy of internal auditory meatus. *VII* Facial nerve, *CO* cochlear nerve, *SV* superior vestibular nerve, *IV* inferior vestibular nerve

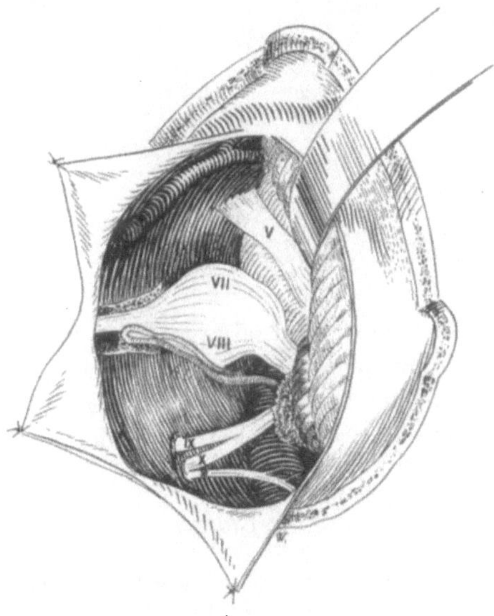

Fig. 15. Appearance of cranial nerves after removal of tumor. Nerves are designated by Roman numerals. Note splaying out of facial and cochlear nerves

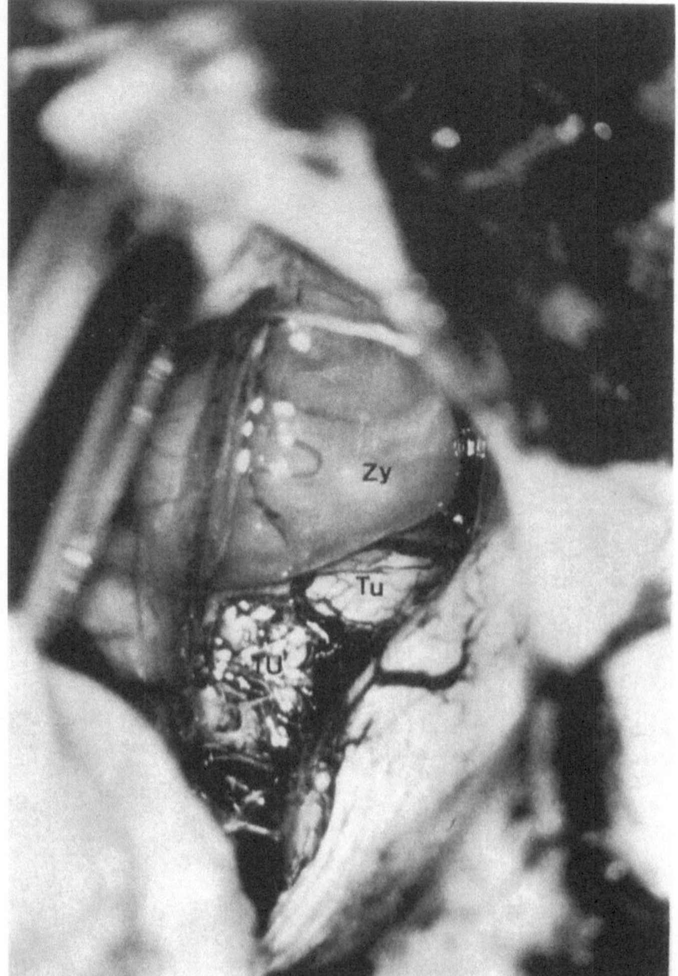

Fig. 16a. Fluid filled cerebellopontine cistern (*Zy*) over tumor (*Tu*)

prevent recurrence the tumor must always be radically removed, so that in these 11 patients this tumor piece was excised and the nerve ends reanastomosed with microsuture. If the tedious freeing of the nerves succeeds, the remaining tumor generally presents no problem (Figs. 15 and 16a–f).

8. *Closure*

After extirpation of the tumor, the tumor bed is rinsed copiously with physiological saline and all bone dust washed from the internal auditory meatus. Before closing the dura, white bone wax (Ethicon, Ltd.) is carefully pressed on all edges of meatus that were drilled and muscle is laid over this and fixed with a bonding agent, Aron Alpha A® (Sankyo Co., Ltd., Japan) to prevent

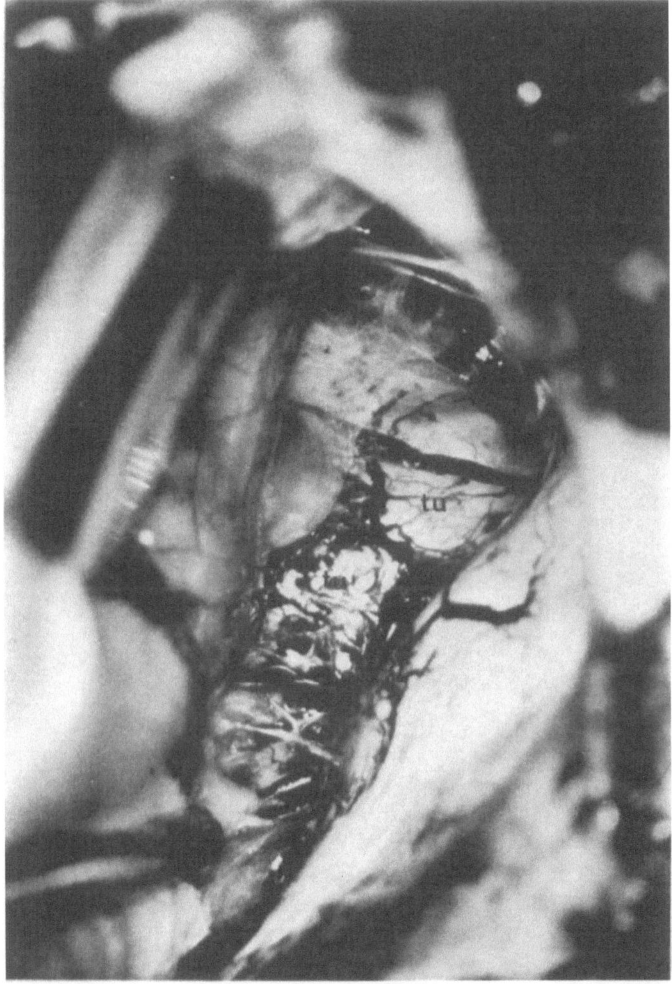

Fig. 16b. After release of xanthochromic fluid from the cistern, the tumor (*tu*) is better visualized

possible cerebrospinal fluid rhinorrhea from leakage into the air cells, middle ear and through the Eustachian tube to the nose.

In some patients the dura could be closed watertight with interrupted or running sutures, but in others because of exceptionally thin dura, tears from retraction or necessary coagulation of dural vessels only approximating sutures could be placed or the dura was simply left open and the opening covered with Tabotamp. The bone flap is replaced and secured with four nylon sutures. The wound is closed in layers. The skin is closed with an atraumatic running nylon suture and sprayed with an adhesive Nobecutan (Bofors, Nobel-Pharma, Sweden). The wound is covered with thin gauze strips held in place by paper tape. The patient is transferred from the operating table to his bed and placed in a half-sitting position (Figs. 17a–d).

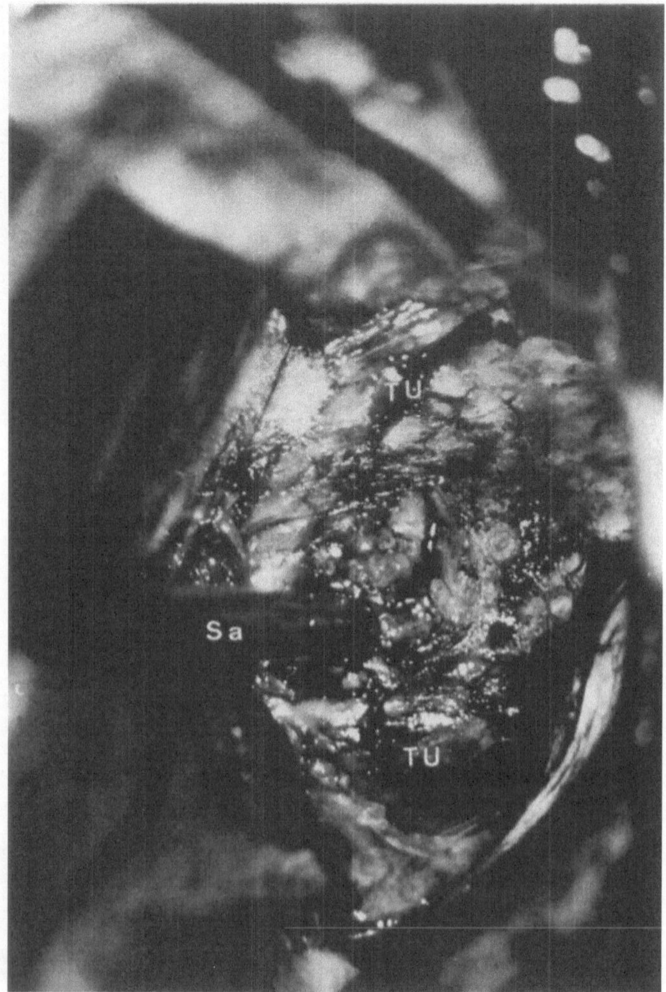

Fig. 16c. Gutting of the tumor. *TU* Tumor, *Sa* sucker

V. Results of Microsurgical Operations on Acoustic Neurinoma

Preoperative grades and postoperative results are summarized in Table 2. Postoperatively 147 patients remain in good to excellent condition (self sufficient and working unless unable to work on account of age). Sixteen patients are considered in fair condition in that they are self sufficient but are no longer able to pursue their usual employment, due either to cerebellar symptoms, tinnitus or facial paresis. Cerebellar symptoms in these patients were for the most part present preoperatively, being noted postoperatively for the first time in only two patients. Four patients require nursing or custodial care and are listed under poor condition. Two of these were unchanged from preoperative status, while two deteriorated postoperatively. Of the latter two one patient underwent operation in the prone position in 1967, wherein a large tumor could

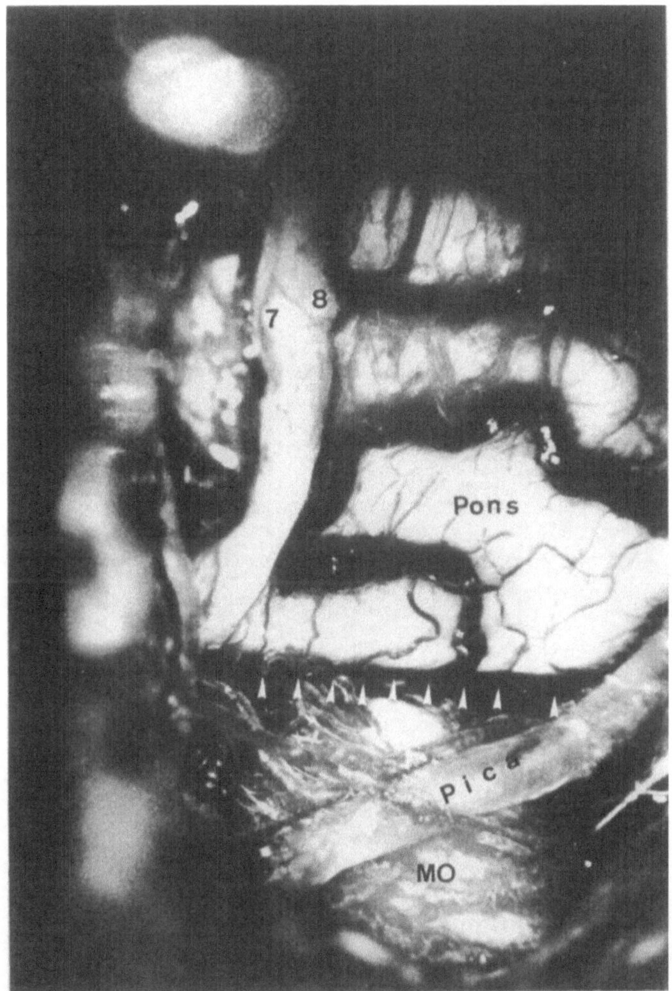

Fig. 16d. Tumor has been removed. Arrows delineate the pontomedullary sulcus. *MO* Medulla oblongata, *7* and *8* facial and cochlear nerves

Table 2. *Acoustic Neurinomas Preoperative Condition and Operative Results* (September 9, 1967 until July 20, 1976)

Preop. grade	No of cases	Good	Fair	Poor	Death
I	24	24 (1)	—	—	—
II	63	61	2	—	—
III	58	50 (4)	5 (2)	2	1
IV	26	12 (2)	9 (3)	2	3 (1)
	171	147	16	4	4

( ) Bilateral tumors = 13.

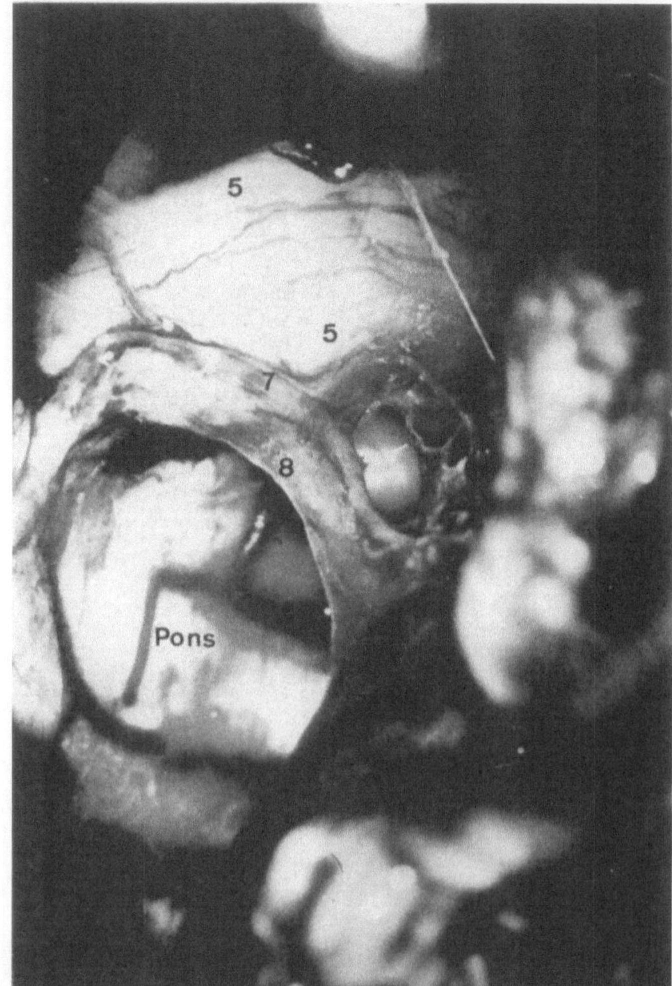

Fig. 16e. Appearance of the facial (*7*) and cochlear (*8*) nerves at the level of the trigeminal nerve (*5*)

not be completely extirpated. He refused further operative intervention and remains crippled with a hemiataxia which does not allow him to leave his home alone. In the second case, acute clinical deterioration occurred 8 days post-operatively. Reexploration revealed thrombosis of the posterior inferior cerebellar artery most probably due to trauma to the artery during extirpation of the tumor. He suffered a lateral-medullary infarction syndrome with a severe hemiataxia and although able to care for himself could no longer continue working. Except for these two patients, no newly occurring hemiparesis or hemiataxia was observed. On the contrary, in most cases pre-existing neurological findings diminished or disappeared within a few weeks to months. New lesions of the trochlear and trigeminal nerves were not observed. Transient paresis of the

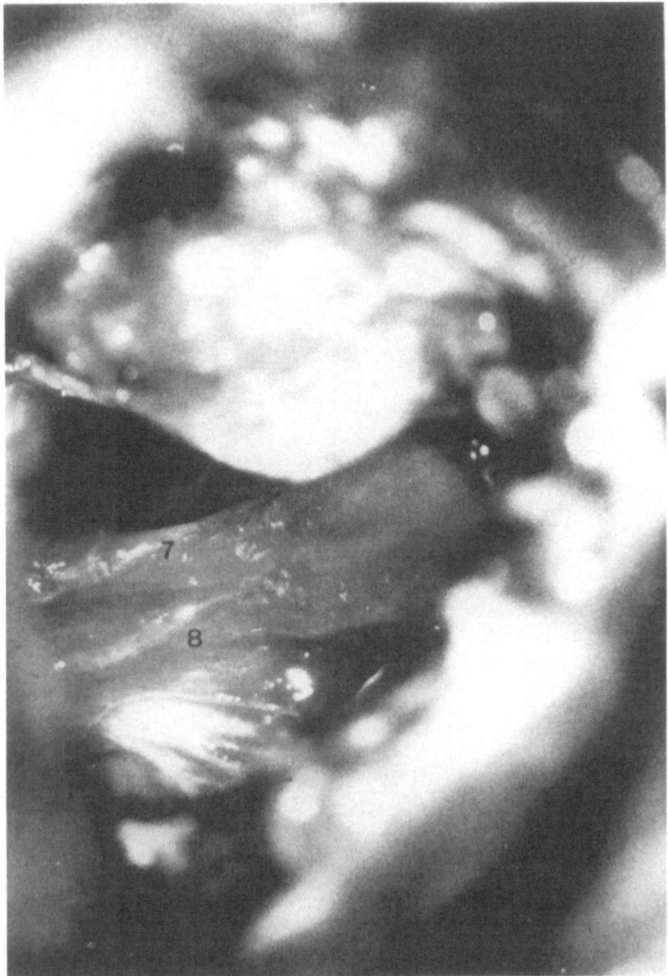

Fig. 16f. Intrameatal portions of the facial (*7*) and cochlear (*8*) nerves

abducens nerve was observed in 4 cases and symptoms referable to partial lesions of nerves IX and X seen in 9 cases.

Four patients died*; a patient with bilateral acoustic neurinomas, a trigeminal neurinoma and a frontal falx meningioma, who was preoperatively in exceedingly poor condition; a 67 year old patient who died of pulmonary embolus 3 months postoperatively; a patient who developed a staphylococcal meningitis 5 months after operation; and a patient who was in grade IV condition preoperatively. The latter patient underwent exploration in the sitting position. With placement of the burr holes it was noted that the dura was very tense, whereupon an occipital burr hole was placed and the occipital horn of the ventricle punctured

* Three cases in 1967, last case December 1972; from 1973 to date no death has occurred in 104 cases.

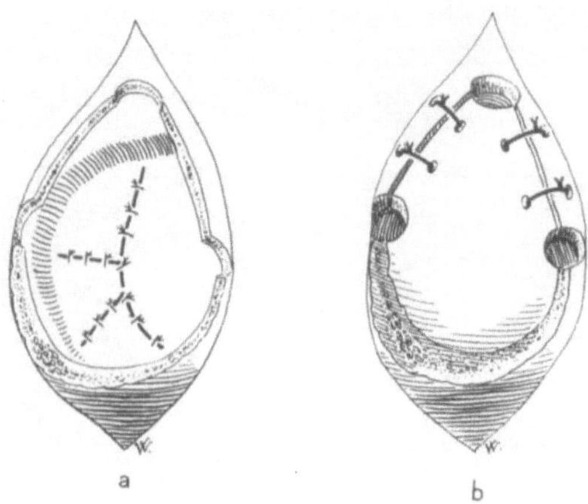

Fig. 17a. Dural closure
Fig. 17b. Replacement of bone flap

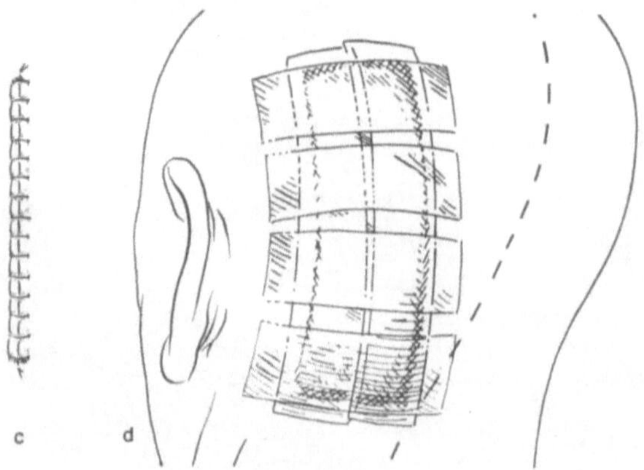

Fig. 17c. Skin closure
Fig. 17d. Application of gauze dressing

to remove cerebrospinal fluid. The patient did not awaken from anesthesia and remained in coma 12 weeks, breathing spontaneously with equal reactive pupils but tetraplegic and unresponsive to pain. At autopsy there were no lesions observed in the pons or medulla, but bandlike softening extended subcortically from the frontal area to the occipital.

1. Function of the Facial Nerve (Table 3)

In 148 patients it was possible to preserve the continuity of the facial nerve. In the postoperative period almost all the patients demonstrated on the second to third day a light to moderate facial paresis involving all branches of the facial nerve which lasted days to few weeks and in some cases even months. After a six months period of observation 114 patients had complete restoration of facial nerve function while 27 showed partial loss of nerve function especially of the nervus intermedius with diminished tear secretion, loss of taste and mimicking movements on the affected side with active closing of the lids or movement of the corner of the mouth. In 137 large tumors only 28 patients showed a facial palsy, despite the fact that in many of these 137 cases the facial nerve was displaced and elongated up to 5 cm and often was widened into a transparent membrane.

Table 3. *Function of Facial Nerve*

Tumor size	No of cases	Anatomically		Function		
		preserved	not preserved	full	partial	no
< 2 cm	4	4	—	2	2	—
2–3 cm	30	29	1	25	3	2
3–5 cm	69	61	8	51	9	9
5 < cm	68	54	14	36	13	19
	171	148	23	114	27	30

Table 4. *Late Results in 30 Patients with VII-Palsy*

Anastomosis	Number of cases	Good	Partial	Unchanged
VII–VII (intracranial)	11	4	5	2
VII–XII (extracranial)	14	6	8	—
Refused	2	—	—	2
Death	3			
	30	10	13	4

Of thirty patients with facial palsy, in eleven patients the facial nerve was intentionally excised in its midportion because the nerve could not be completely separated from the tumor and a complete extirpation was felt necessary. The cut ends of the facial nerve were anastomosed with two microsutures. Four patients showed complete recovery of facial nerve function after one year and 5 others had partial improvement. In two patients the end result has not been determined because the period of observation has not extended to 6 months. In the other 19 cases, the origin and meatal portions of the nerve remained intact over a length of about one centimeter but the middle portion could not be dissected free and saved, leaving too great a gap for primary anastomosis. Three patients in this group died before a facial-hypoglossal nerve anastomosis could be performed and two patients refused this operation. The 14 remaining patients underwent facial-hypoglossal nerve anastomosis in the otorhinolaryngology clinic at the University of Zurich and the results of these operations are shown in Table 4.

2. Function of the Cochlear Nerve

In 40% of cases it was possible to dissect the cochlear nerve free of tumor capsule, however in only one case was objective hearing function preserved. In this case a 2 centimeter tumor had minimal adherence to the nerves. In another five cases there was a slight degree of hearing function for a few days postoperatively which gradually disappeared to be replaced by tinnitus. One of these cases required re-exploration and division of the cochlear nerve because of the degree of tinnitus. Other cases of postoperative tinnitus spontaneously abated. Preservation of hearing is a point increasingly emphasized in recent discussions.

3. Complications

a) Hematoma

In four cases postoperative hematoma occurred. These were epidural, subdural, intracerebellar and in the tumor bed.

b) Thrombosis of the Posterior Inferior Cerebellar Artery

As was described above this unusual complication was observed in one patient on the eighth postoperative day.

c) Infection

Many patients showed a transient temperature elevation in the postoperative period generally in the range of 38–39 °C. Bacteriological examination revealed Staphylococcal infection in 6 cases and Klebsiella in one. All patients were given Chloramphenicol (Chloromycetin®, Parke-Davis, U.S.A.) prophylactically—2 grams daily in the pre- and postoperative periods. The patients with positive bacteriological culture and sensitivity determinations were treated with the indicated antibiotic, for the most part Cefalothin (Keflin®, Lilly, U.S.A.), 12 gms., and Garamycin® (Schering Corp., U.S.A.) 240 mgs. per day. It would be inappropriate to discuss the more chronic infections such as cystitis, pneumonia or phlebitis and pulmonary embolism in detail. Thirty per cent of patients, generally those in preoperative Grades III and IV had some indication of postoperative infection while the other 70% had unremarkable postoperative courses and were discharged home 10–14 days after operation.

d) Disturbances in Cerebrospinal Fluid Circulation

Earlier patients (until 1973) in this series had a ventriculo-atrial shunt placed if signs of increased intracranial pressure such as papilledema or diminished level of consciousness were present preoperatively (14 cases). Later it has not been felt necessary to perform preoperative shunting of these patients and no significant difficulty at operation has been noted.

Twelve patients required a postoperative ventriculo-atrial shunt for communicating hydrocephalus. These were done weeks to months after operation and frequently resulted in dramatic abatement of cerebellar symptoms.

Thirtyeight patients developed subgaleal cerebrospinal fluid collections which were often quite persistant. Development of a subgaleal fluid collection did not depend on the tightness of the dural closure or the replacement of the bone flap although the latter improved cosmetic effect. A disturbance in cerebrospinal fluid pathways and resorption seemed to be the origin of these collections. Patients were treated by lumbar puncture, head elevation, compressive bandages and eight cases ventriculo-atrial shunts. Computerized axial tomography may provide a convenient way to follow these fluid collections and the development of hydrocephalus.

e) Cerebrospinal Fluid Rhinorrhea

Seven patients developed cerebrospinal fluid rhinorrhea in the postoperative period. In two cases this ceased spontaneously after 4–6 weeks while in the remaining 5 cases reexploration was required. In two patients the fistula was found in the mastoid air cells and in the other three in the drilled area of the internal auditory meatus where the bone had been inadequately sealed with wax. Successful closure of the fistula was achieved in all cases.

f) Tinnitus

Tinnitus present preoperatively generally disappeared or diminished after the operation. In one patient postoperative tinnitus was intolerable such that she required a second procedure to sever the cochlear nerve which had been painstakingly preserved at the first operation.

VI. Bilateral Acoustic Neurinoma

The following discussion is based on 13 cases; 8 patients were afflicted with neurofibromatosis, with bilateral cranial nerve tumors, not only on the vestibular nerve but also on the trigeminal nerve (3 cases), abducens nerve (1 case), facial nerve (2 cases), the glossopharyngeal and vagus nerves (5 cases), the spinal accessory nerve (2 cases), and the hypoglossal nerve (1 case). Two of these patients also had multiple spinal neurinomas and one other had frontal bilateral falx meningiomas. Five cases had only bilateral acoustic neurinomas without other signs of neurofibromatosis. It is technically possible to extirpate bilateral tumors at one operation. It is however not possible to give a definite prognosis regarding postoperative function of the facial and especially the cochlear nerves. Therefore the indications for bilateral exploration whether at one or two operations are very difficult to evaluate, especially when the patient demonstrates good hearing on one side.

In five cases a large acoustic neurinoma had already been subtotally removed on one side in another hospital. All these patients demonstrated hearing loss and facial weakness on that side. Progressive symptomatology of a tumor on the opposite side forced a second operation, and in no case could residual hearing present preoperatively be saved so that all 5 cases remained deaf postoperatively. The facial nerves were saved and these later showed good facial function.

A 25-year-old female patient with neurofibromatosis had in addition to an acoustic neurinoma a large trigeminal neurinoma and a bilateral frontal falx meningioma. Preoperatively she was blind and deaf and because of breathing and swallowing difficulty had a tracheotomy performed. At the insistence of the family the patient was operated on in Grade IV condition through a combined translabyrinthine and suboccipital approach. It was not possible to completely remove the tumors because the acoustic neurinoma had infiltrated the petrous bone and the trigeminal neurinoma filled the middle fossa. The patient died six days after operation [first case of the senior author (MGY)].

A 15-year-old girl had clinical and radiological findings suggesting a large acoustic neurinoma on one side and a smaller tumor on the other side. It was therefore decided to carry out bilateral cerebellopontine angle exploration at one operation. Surprisingly at the operation she was found to have large acoustic neurinomas bilaterally, and additional small tumors along the glossopharyngeal, vagus and spinal accessory nerves and on one side a trigeminal neurinoma. She withstood the operation well and postoperatively had no facial weakness although she had no residual hearing.

In a 24-year-old female with neurofibromatosis, bilateral acoustic neurinomas and bilateral frontal falx meningiomas were diagnosed by clinical and radiographic signs. The right-sided acoustic neurinoma was operated on first because that was the side with least hearing. Postoperatively the patient had a permanent facial weakness although the facial nerve was anatomically intact at the operation. One year later a facial-hypoglossal nerve anastomosis was performed. The patient had learned in the meantime to read and use sign language, and she underwent a second operation 2½ years after the first. Exploration revealed multiple neurinomas on cranial nerves VIII, IX, X, XI, and XII in addition to a large cerebellopontine angle meningioma which covered the neurinomas like a cap. A left sided intramedullary cyst was also found although the patient had shown no bulbar or pyramidal tract signs. Facial nerve function remained intact postoperatively but the patient required a tracheotomy for swallowing difficulty. She recovered quickly from her operation and is now well.

In five other patients with bilateral tumors, exploration was carried out only on the side with the greatest hypacusis and the tumor was completely removed. The opposite tumor was not attacked because worthwhile hearing function remained.

From the above described examples it is clear that an all-inclusive surgical dictum cannot be given for patients with bilateral or multiple tumors. Each case must be considered individually. One must determine how long the patient has had his complaints and symptoms and how many operations can be reasonably performed.

VII. Anesthesia

The following monitoring devices are employed on patients undergoing operation of acoustic neurinoma:

1. A four lead electrocardiograph.

2. Continuous recording of arterial blood pressure through a cannula inserted in the radial artery. The transducer is placed at the level of the cranium to insure cerebral arterial pressure is adequate.

3. A catheter is placed in the right atrium either through a subclavian vein puncture or through an antecubital vein. Chest roentgenography verifies the position of the catheter and checks for pneumothorax where subclavian puncture has been performed. Intravascular electrocardiography is also used to assess catheter placement.

4. A Doppler apparatus over the precordium to detect air embolism.

5. A rectal thermistor.

6. A mirror mounted at face level if the patient is turned away from the anesthesiologist. This allows the anesthesiologist to report the result of intraoperative facial nerve stimulation (see Fig. 2c).

The patients legs are wrapped in elastic bandages to avoid venous pooling.

One half hour prior to intubation, patients are given Innovar® (Janssen Pharmaceutica, Belgium), a combination of Fentanyl® and Droperidol (Dehydrobenzperidol®), 0.2 ml/kg and atropine sulfate, 0.01 mg/kg intramuscularly. For induction with general anesthesia an anti-fascicular dose of Pancuronium (Pavulon®, Organon, Holland), 0.5 mg/kg, Droperidol (Dehydrobenzperidol®, Janssen Pharmaceutica, Belgium), 0.1 mg/kg, Fentanyl®, 0.005 mg/kg, and a sleep dose of Methohexital (Brietal Sodium®, Lilly, U.S.A.), 0.75 mg/kg are given intravenously. The patient is manually ventilated with one hundred per cent oxygen and paralyzed with Succinylcholine (Celocuoin®, Vitrum, Sweden), 1 mg/kg for oral intubation. Mechanical ventilation with an Engström Respirator with a 2 : 1 mixture of Nitrous oxide to oxygen is started, and adequate ventilation is checked by arterial blood gas analysis. A positive end-expiratory pressure (PEEP) of + 8 cm H_2O is utilized to prevent air embolism, and if air embolism occurs the anesthesiologist compresses the jugular veins to allow the surgeon to detect open veins in the operating field.

Anesthesia is maintained with intravenous doses of Fentanyl®. Orthostatic hypotension following the sitting positioning is corrected with Dextran (Macrodex®, Pharmacia) or gelatine solutions. Hypertensive episodes caused by stimulation of the trigeminal nerve are treated with Enflurane (Ethrane®, Abbott, U.S.A.) or Halothan® (Hoechst, Westgermany), (1–2%) over a short period. Bradycardia secondary to stimulation of the vagus nerve is treated with intravenous atropine sulfate.

VIII. Conclusion

Surgery of acoustic neurinoma has advanced from a stage where only intracapsular removal of the tumor was deemed feasible to a stage where the most modern technical advancements are employed for complete extirpation of the tumor and preservation of the facial nerve. Better understanding of the pathological anatomy, remarkable improvements in radiological techniques, and use of the operating microscope and microsurgical technique have all contributed to the more favorable prognosis that can now be given to these patients. While it is hoped that earlier diagnosis and treatment will result in further improvements, it is anticipated that for several years large acoustic neurinomas will require the skill of neurosurgeons. Experience with microsurgical technique has shown that even the largest tumors can be totally removed through a small craniotomy with only minimal retraction of the cerebellar hemisphere. With piecemeal evacuation of the tumor parenchyma, the tumor tends to collapse inward allowing accurate dissection of the capsule from the neural and vascular structures. With the above described technique for operative management of an acoustic neurinoma, the operating microscope is utilized from the time of the craniotomy until the dura has been closed. A detailed presentation of this operative technique of the senior author (M. G. Y.) has been given and the results of his 171 patients evaluated.

References

Cushing, H., 1917: Tumors of nervus acusticus and syndrome of cerebello-pontine angle. Philadelphia: W. B. Saunders Company.

Dandy, W. E., 1941: Results of removal of acoustic tumors by the unilateral approach. A. M. A. Arch. Surg. *42*, 1026—1033.

De Martel, T., 1931: Surgical treatment of cerebral tumors. Technical considerations. Surg. Gynec. Obstet. *52*, 381—385.

Di Chiro, G., 1967: An atlas of pathologic pneumoencephalographic anatomy. Springfield, Ill.: Ch. C Thomas.

Drake, C. G., 1967: Surgical treatment of acoustic neuroma with preservation or reconstruction of the facial nerve. J. Neurosurg. *26*, 459—464.

— 1967: Total removal of large acoustic neurinomas. A modification of the McKenzie operation with special emphasis on saving the facial nerve. J. Neurosurg. *26*, 554—561.

Epstein, B. S., 1966: Pneumoencephalography and cerebral angiography. In: Year Book Medical Publ., Chicago, p. 1—17.

Fay, T., 1931: The management of tumors of the posterior fossa by the transtentorial approach. Surg. Clin. H. Amer. *10*, 14 —27.

Fisch, U., 1968: L'anatomie chirurgicale du système artériel du conduit auditif interne chez l'homme. Rev. Laryng. (Bordeaux) *89*, 11, 12, 659—671.

— Weber, J., 1972: Der diagnostische Wert der Pantopaque-Cisternographie. Méd. Hyg. *30*, 1567—1568.

Hitselberger, W. E., Raney, A. A., 1964: Neurosurgical thoughts comparing suboccipital and translabyrinthine approaches. Arch. Otolaryng. (Chicago) *80/6*, 754—756.

— House, W. F., 1966: A combined approach to the cerebellopontine angle: a suboccipital-petrosal approach. Arch. Otolaryng. (Chicago) *84*, 267—285.

House, W. F., 1961: Surgical exposure of the internal auditory canal and its contents through the middle cranial fossa. Laryngoscope *11*, 1363—1385.

Key, A., Retzius, G., 1875: Studien in der Anatomie des Nervensystems und des Bindegewebes. Stockholm: Verlag Samson & Wallin.

Kümmel, W., 1909: Otologische Gesichtspunkte bei der Diagnose und Therapie von Erkrankungen der hinteren Schädelgrube. Deutsch. Z. Nervenheilk. *36*, 132—142.

Kurze, T., Doyle, J. B., 1962: Extradural intracranial (middle fossa) approach to the internal auditory canal. J. Neurosurg. *19*, 1033—1077.

Leighton, R. S., 1971: Neuroradiologic anatomy. A stereoscopic atlas. Baltimore: The Williams & Wilkins Company.

Liliequist, B., 1959: The subarachnoid cisterns. Anatomic and roentgenologic study. Acta Radiol. Suppl. 185, Stockholm.

— 1959: Pontine angle tumor. Encephalographic appearances. Acta Radiol. Suppl. 186, Stockholm.

McClure Wilson, 1972: The anatomical foundation of neurology of the brain subarachnoid spaces, Chapter 4, pp. 93—103. Boston: Little Brown. 1963.

McKenzie, K. G., Alexander, E., 1955: Acoustic neurinoma. Clin. Neurosurg. *2*, 21—36.

Morrison, A. W., King, T. T., 1973: Experiences with a translabyrinthine-transtentorial approach to the cerebellopontine angle. Technical note. J. Neurosurg. *38*, 382—390.

Olivecrona, H., 1940: Acoustic tumors. J. Neurosurg. Psychiat. *3*, 141—146.

— 1967: The surgical treatment of intracranial tumors. 1. Meningiomas of posterior surface of the petrous bone, pp. 181—184. 2. The neurinomas, pp. 192—222. In: Handbuch der Neurochirurgie, Bd. 4, 4. Teil (Olivecrona, H., Tönnis, W., Ed.). Berlin-Heidelberg-New York: Springer.

Panse, R., 1904: Ein Gliom des Akustikus. Arch. Ohr. *61*, 251—255.

Pertuiset, B. *et al.*, 1970: Les neurinomes de l'acoustique, développés dans l'angle ponto-cérébelleux. Neuro-Chir. 1, Suppl. 1, 16.

Pool, J. L., Pava, A. A., 1957: The early diagnosis and treatment of acoustic nerve tumors, p. 161. Springfield, Ill.: Ch. C Thomas.

Portmann, M., Sterkers, J. M., Charachon, R., Chouard, Ch., Bebear, J.-P., Junien-Lavillauroy, C., Pelisse, J. M., Peytral, C., 1973: Anatomie, pathologie et chirurgie du conduit auditif interne. Paris: Arnette éd.

Quix, F. H., 1911: Ein Acusticustumor. In: III. Niederländische Gesellschaft für Hals-, Nasen- und Ohrenheilkunde. Arch. Ohr.-Nas.-Kehlkopfheilk. *84*, 252—253.

Rand, R. W., Kurze, T., 1965: Microneurosurgical resection of acoustic tumors by a transmeatal posterior fossa approach. Bull. Los Ang. Neurol. Soc. *30*, 17—20.

Rosomoff, H. L., 1971: The subtemporal transtentorial approach to the cerebellopontine angle. Laryngoscope *81*, 1448—1454.

Samii, M., 1974: Pneumoenzephalo-Tomographie. Stuttgart: F. Enke.

Schmiegelow, E., 1915: Beitrag zur translabyrinthinen Entfernung der Akustikustumoren. Z. Ohrenheilk. *93*, 1—21.

Yaşargil, M. G., 1976: Subokzipitale-transmeatale mikrotechnische Exstirpation des Akustikusneurinomes. In: Kopf- und Hals-Chirurgie, Bd. 3, pp. 545—587 (Hrsg. H. H. Naumann). Stuttgart: G. Thieme.

Zange, J., 1915: Translabyrinthäre Operationen von Acusticus- und Kleinhirnbrückenwinkeltumoren. Klin. Wschr. *52*, 1334.

Balloon Arterial Catheter Techniques in the Treatment of Arterial Intracranial Diseases

G. Debrun, P. Lacour, and J. P. Caron

University Hospital Henri Mondor, Department of Neuro-Radiology and Neuro-Surgery, Créteil (France)

With 17 Figures

Contents

Carotid-cavernous fistulas treatment by a balloon released in the cavernous sinus, and preserving carotid flow, was first performed by Serbinenko[1] and has raised intense interest.

Our own technique of inflatable and releasable balloons has already been described[2–5]. A more detailed presentation of this technique and of its applications is the purpose of this paper.

Making the Latex Sleeve

By dipping stainless steel moulds in pure latex, one obtains small latex finger shaped sleeves used for balloon production; the shape and the size of the mould determines that of the sleeves (Fig. 1): mould diameter varies from 0.2 to one millimeter; a sleeve of 0.2 millimeter diameter will give an inflated balloon of 0.3 centimeter. In order to obtain bigger balloons, one uses a one millimeter diameter mould, with a spherical tip 2 or 3 millimeters in diameter. These balloons can be inflated to a diameter of two to four centimeters, sufficient for the treatment of the biggest aneurysms.

After dipping into latex, the moulds are put in an oven, and steam treated at 100 °C for half an hour; the sleeves are then slipped off.

Making the Balloon

If we want to see the balloon fluoroscopically without injection of contrast, we can put a silver clip inside the latex sleeve. The end of the sleeve must be ligated over the clip.

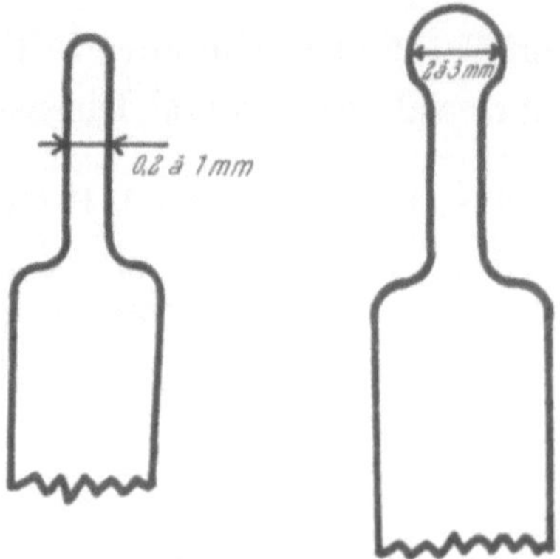

Fig. 1. Different shapes of stainless steel moulds

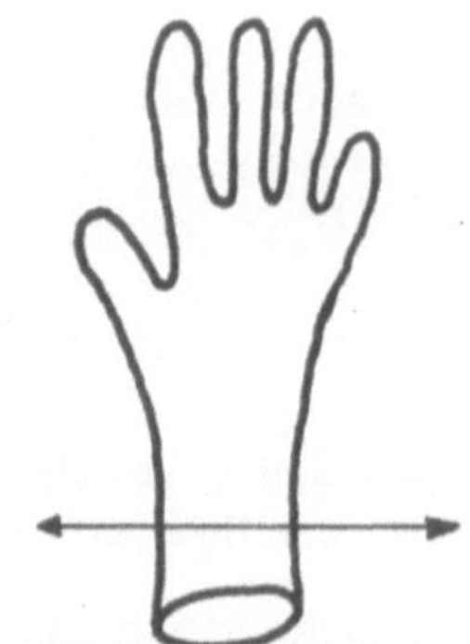

Fig. 2. The elastic thread is cut off from a latex glove as shown by the arrow

Manufacture of the balloon is accomplished by pulling the sleeve over a first catheter* which will be called A. The deeper the catheter A is pushed into the sleeve, the smaller the balloon will be.

The sleeve is then tied onto the catheter A with a thin elastic thread cut from a latex glove in the axis of the glove (Fig. 2): this is accomplished by one person holding the catheter A and the sleeve at the proper distance from the end of the sleeve, while another person prepares a knot with the latex thread, and secures it over the sleeve as near as possible to the fingers of the first person (Fig. 3).

The balloon is then inflated and the second person takes eight half turns with each end of the rubber thread: thus in all (including the first knot), the thread is

* B.D. 7608 ⌀ 0.25/0.51 mm or lymphography catheter by Biotrol France 1, rue du Foin 75140 Paris Cedex 3, No. 1, ⌀ 0.3/0.7 mm or Teflon B.D. No. 6426, ⌀ 0.38/0.69 mm.

wound around the catheter A five times. On the last loop, three simple knots are made (Fig. 4). The different loops should not overlap. The two ends of the thread are cut as near as possible to the knot, with thin scissors. No magnifying glass nor microscope is required.

The part of the sleeve which is not to be used is cut off as close as possible to the ligature (Fig. 5).

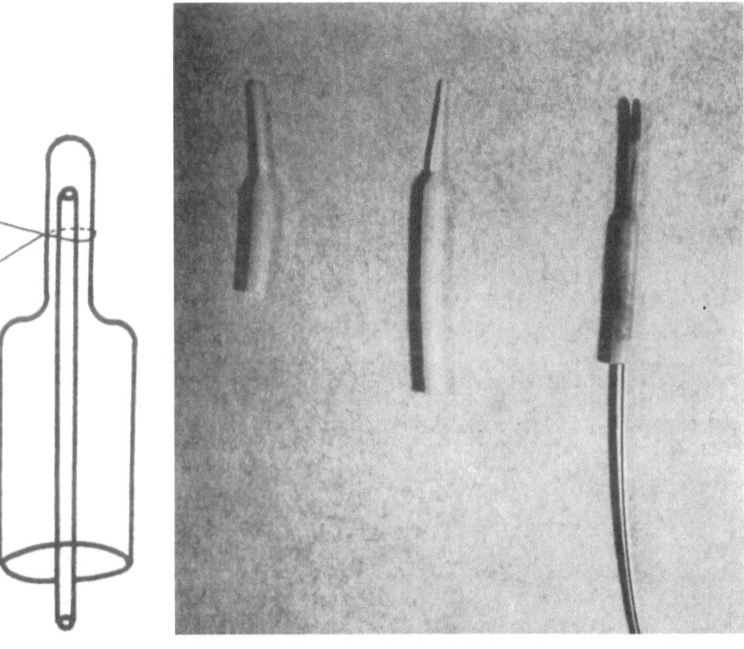

Fig. 3 a Fig. 3 b

Manufacture of the balloons and their ligature on the catheter A are performed on the day of their use, to avoid loss of elasticity of the rubber thread.

In order to facilitate the release of the balloon, the tip of the catheter A is lubricated with vaseline oil before pulling the sleeve over it. Silicone must not be used for this purpose, since it is too slippery.

To ensure that the balloon is not released unintentionally the ligature on the catheter A must be tight. This does make the release of the balloon more difficult.

Release of the balloon is obtained by mean of a second co-axial catheter B, which is slipped over the first catheter A and pushes the balloon off; for this, the internal diameter of the catheter B* must be very close to the external diameter of the catheter A.

* Radiopaque polyéthylène Ingenor-Surgimed No. 15 catheter, is used over the B.D. 7608 catheter; Ingenor-Surgimed No. 14 is used with Biotrol No. 1; Ingenor-Surgimed No. 15 is used over teflon B.D. No. 6426, which must be straightened until it enters Surgimed No. 15.

The outer catheter B keeps the balloon in the proper position, when the inner catheter A is pulled out to release the balloon (Fig. 6). The balloon aperture is immediately closed by the elasticity of the rubber thread, thus avoiding leakage.

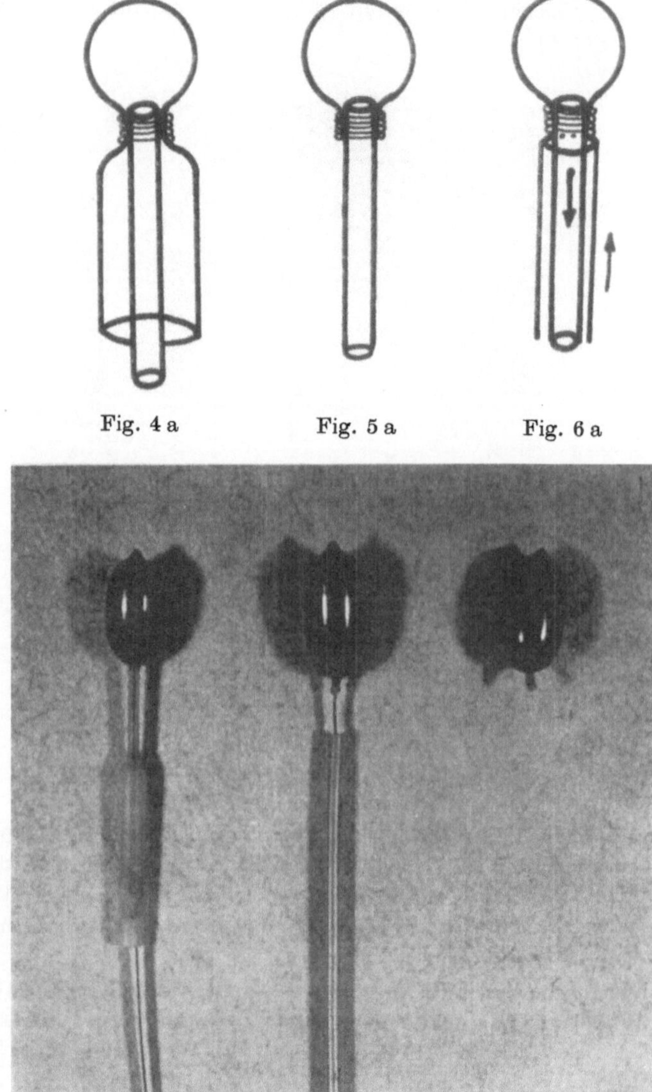

Fig. 4 a Fig. 5 a Fig. 6 a

Fig. 4 b Fig. 5 b Fig. 6 b

The stress exerted by the ligature on the catheter A is empirical but very critical. If this ligature is too tight, withdrawal of the catheter A may become difficult or even impossible, and there is a risk of breaking the catheter. The use of teflon for the inner catheter A would help to avoid this short-coming, but teflon on the other hand is rigid. If the ligature is not tight enough, the balloon may be released too early, or leakage may occur when an iodine-based contrast medium is used. Replacement of the iodine-contrast by a polymerizing mixture solves this problem, as the balloon will keep its volume permanently. Much practice is required for the technique to become reliable, and it is essential to practice making the catheters.

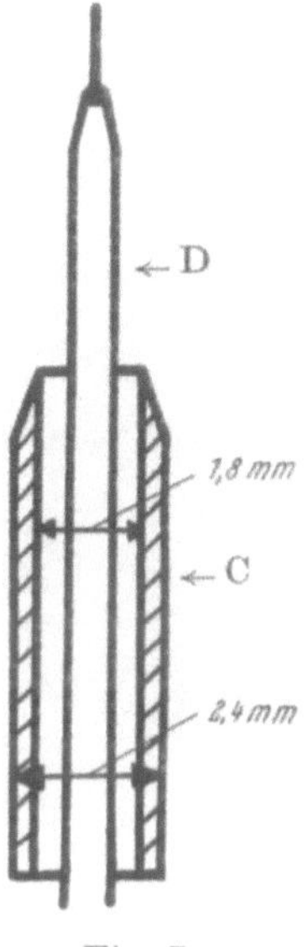

Fig. 7

Balloons inflated with contrast can be released without any immediate leakage, but experience has shown that often balloons become smaller after a fortnight; a second balloon was necessary for two patients. For this reason, iodine contrast is now replaced by a liquid which sets in ten minutes.

Introducing the Catheters into the Carotid Artery

Both inner (A) and outer (B) catheter (and the attached balloon) are introduced into the internal carotid artery by means of an introducer "C", 1.8 mm inside diameter, 2.4 mm outside diameter (Ingenor No. 7666); this catheter C is placed according to Seldinger's technique, modified as explained below (Fig. 7)[6].

The common carotid artery is catheterized with a 18 T needle; a 160 guide is introduced into the common carotid artery and then into the external carotid artery, to avoid any endarterial lesion of the internal carotid artery.

An Ingenor-Surgimed No. 13 (⌀ 0.14/1.50 mm catheter) (D) is first introduced on this guide, followed by the final Ingenor 7666 catheter which is called "the introducer C".

This introduction is carried out under television control; the introducer C is then pulled back into the common carotid artery and brought into the internal carotid artery at C 2–C 3 level, with a flexible 160 guide with a curved tip. The internal diameter of the introducer C must be wide enough to allow the passage of the outer co-axial catheter B, continuous isotonic glucose infusion and iodine

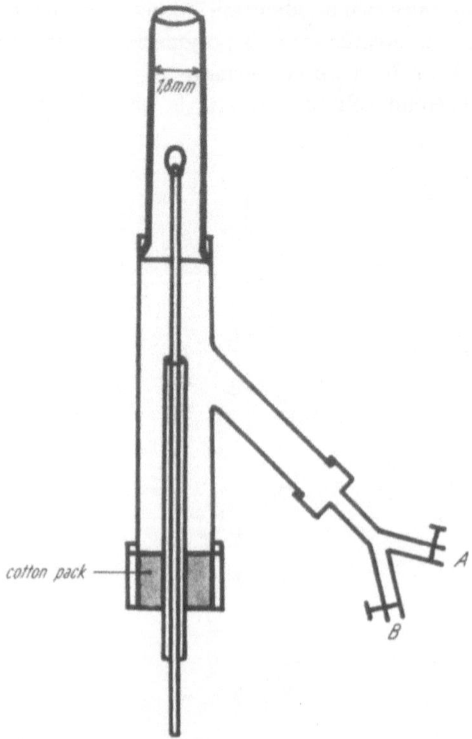

Fig. 8. *A*: Heparinised perfusion, *B*: Contrast

contrast injection; this permanent infusion (Fig. 8 *B*) and iodine contrast injection for peroperative angiographic controls (Fig. 8 *A*) are made possible by using a λ shaped pipe which is attached to the rear end of the introducer C.

The penetration of the introducer C into the carotid wall can be difficult, especially if the carotid artery has already been punctured a few days earlier; in such a case, a Cordis vessel dilator* is first introduced in the carotid artery along the guide, before the two Ingenor catheters are inserted.

The co-axial catheter B and the balloon catheter A can then be passed through the straight part of the λ shaped pipe (Fig. 8); loss of blood along the co-axial catheter B is prevented by a seal made of soaked cotton with heparinised jelly; this is packed into the nut at the bottom of the λ shaped pipe. The inner catheter A is twenty centimeters longer than the co-axial catheter B; this extra length of the inner catheter A is used to place the balloon in the position where it is to be released.

The operator knows that the co-axial catheter B is in contact with the balloon, when he has pushed it up along the inner catheter A so that twenty centimeters of this last one protrude at his proximal end (Fig. 9). He must measure it before release: it is the only security to be sure that the catheter B has reached the base of the balloon.

---

* Vessel dilator No. 501–200, Cordis, Miami, Florida 33 137.

The operator should also take note that he will not be able to visualise the balloon while it is in the λ shaped pipe and in the introducer C; only after it has reached beyond the introducer C, can it be made visible by iodine contrast injection. Therefore, the total length of the introducer C and λ shaped pipe must be carefully measured.

To get around this difficulty, a silver clip can be put inside the balloon during its manufacture; this clip can be observed radiologically even when it is inside the introducer C. When the balloon has left the introducer C, carotid blood flow

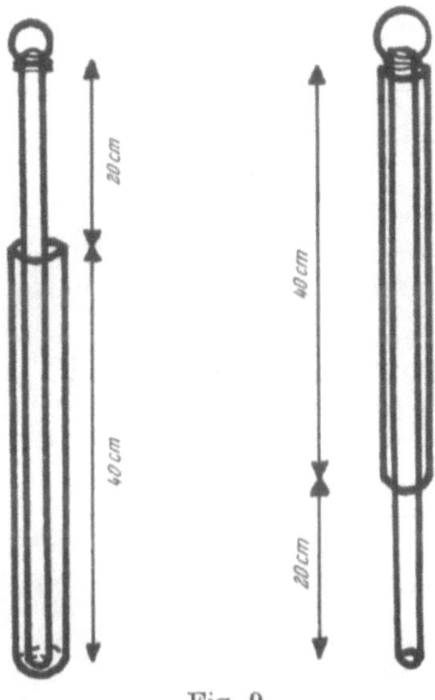

Fig. 9

and the thrust applied to the catheter A are enough to drive the balloon into the carotid siphon.

In some cases, a small iodine injection into the balloon shows it to be at the end of the internal carotid artery. But in other cases, glucose infusion by the lateral foot of the λ shaped pipe is necessary to help the progression of the balloon. One must also know that internal carotid artery kinking can be a major handicap to the progression of the balloon and can even lead to a total failure of the technique if we must reach over the carotid siphon. It may be the case when there is a complete loop of the internal carotid in the neck or when the origin of the internal carotid artery is perpendicular to the common carotid. In this last case it is more careful to expose surgically the origin of the internal carotid.

Indications

The ease with which the balloon is sucked into a carotid-cavernous fistula or toward the arterio-venous shunt of an angioma, contrasts with the difficulty of making the balloon enter an aneurysmal cavity.

For these reasons, good indications for this technique are post-traumatic carotid-cavernous fistulas, and the infrequent vertebro-vertebral fistulas.

Angiomas are not a good indication: obstruction of feeding arterial pedicles far from the angioma, albeit easy, is inefficient. Because of difficulties and hazard of this technique in treatment of aneurysms, it must be used with great care, each case being discussed between the neuro-surgeon and the neuro-radiologist.

Such a possible indication would be presence of an aneurysm on the carotid arterial siphon, the bifurcation of the internal carotid artery, or at the origin of the posterior communicating artery; when the aneurysm is saccular, preferably round, when its neck is from 2 to 5 mm wide, and when there is no associated spasm.

On the other hand, guiding the balloon to anterior communicating artery aneurysms is very difficult. Basilar arterial system aneurysms are very difficult to treat through the femoral artery: the direct puncture of the vertebral artery at the level of its entrance into the skull would be of great help but such a puncture is notoriously dangerous.

For aneurysm treatment, a flexible straight catheter A is usually not convenient; to enter the aneurysm cavity, a teflon catheter A should be used, the tip of which has been pre-operatively bent, after a careful study of the position of the neck of the aneurysm.

None of those difficulties are encountered when the treatment concerns a post-traumatic carotid-cavernous fistula. Definitive clinical cure without impairment of the internal carotid blood flow can be achieved sufficiently often and sufficiently easily to consider henceforth unadvisable the use of the Fogarty catheter for that type of lesion.

Treatment of a Carotid-Cavernous Fistula

The detailed technique of treatment of such a fistula, with the help of a releasable balloon inflated with polymerizing substance, will now be presented. The first step consists in a thorough study of the location of the fistula by means of subtraction X-ray seriographic films, at least 4 to five films per second. Cine-radiography can be quite useful.

Contra-lateral carotid arteriography, as well as vertebral arteriogram, with and without compression of the feeding carotid artery, are requested in order to determine hemodynamic characteristics of the fistula and to know if blood supply to the cerebral hemisphere on the side of the fistula can be insured by anastomosis via the circle of Willis in case it becomes necessary to cut off carotid flow on the side of the fistula. The exact level of the fistula is often determined by these special angiographies.

The goal of the treatment must be to bring the balloon into the cavernous sinus on the venous side of the fistula, to inflate the balloon until the fistula has disappeared on control angiograms, while carotid blood flow is preserved.

After the introducer C has been placed in the internal carotid, the air in the catheter A carrying the balloon is displaced by 0.10 to 0.15 ml of water soluble iodine contrast* (Ioxitalamate de monoéthanolamine + Ioxitalamate de méthylglucamine); a few manœuvers are necessary to get rid of the last air bubble.

* Vasobrix 32, Laboratoires Guerbet, F 93 Aulnay s/bois.

(The aim is to direct the air bubble unto the end of the catheter A and aspirate the bubble while the balloon is still full of contrast.) Then, the balloon catheter A is introduced in the carotid artery and profile radioscopic views control its progression, 0.04 to 0.05 ml of iodine contrast are enough.

Its progression through the dense mastoïd is difficult to observe and television subtraction with videorecording is of assistance. As soon as the balloon has progressed beyond the intra-petrous canal, it is again quite easy to observe. When it reaches the carotid siphon, it tends to be sucked up by the fistula and a slight flutter or a directionnal change indicates to the operator that it has entered

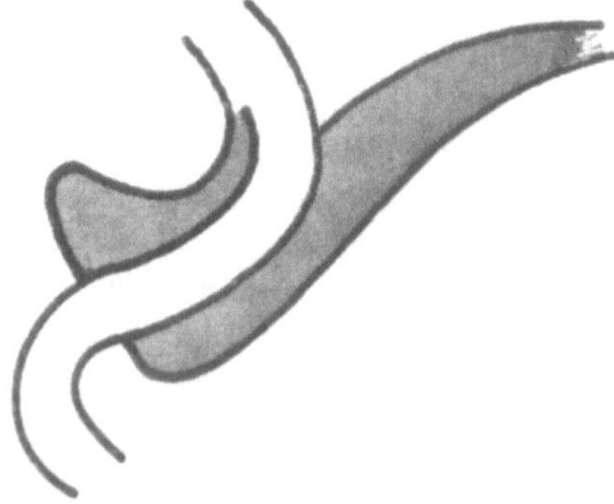

Fig. 10. Carotid-cavernous fistula by a dissection of the internal carotid artery; the fistula aperture is so located that it makes the balloon introduction into it impossible

the cavernous sinus. When the balloon does not quickly enter the cavernous sinus, it should be kept in the neighbourhood of the supposed position of the fistula; small to and fro motions should be applied to the catheter, combined with variations of balloon volume. If this is not successful, the balloon and inner catheter A should be replaced by a smaller balloon.

When the balloon is properly placed inside the cavernous sinus, it must be inflated with about 0.20 ml of iodine contrast and the tap closed. Preservation of the carotid blood flow is then verified by carotid injection of contrast medium, as well as the closure of the fistula. The result is then confirmed by AP and lateral fast seriographic angiograms (four exposures per second during the first three seconds, one per second up to the tenth second, one more at the twelvth, fourteenth and sixteenth second). Any abnormality (leakage of contrast into the cavernous sinus or irregularity in the carotid blood flow) implies that the amount of contrast in the balloon should be modified until perfect conditions obtained.

Because of the location or the narrowness of the fistula (Fig. 10), all the above procedures may fail; in this case, the balloon should be released in the carotid artery, opposite the neck of the fistula, thus plugging the carotid artery.

Final Release of the Balloon

Once the final position has been achieved, the balloon is deflated and the iodine contrast volume that it contained is carefully measured. Part of the contrast remaining in the inner catheter A can not be removed. This volume will have been carefully determined before the balloon is manufactured; the B.D. 7608 catheter (inside ∅ 0.25 mm length 60 cm) will contain 0.05 ml iodine contrast, the Biotrol No. 1 catheter (inside ⌀ 0.30 mm length 60 cm) will contain 0.07 ml. This volume must be known, since it will be reintroduced into the balloon when the polymerizing substance is injected. The polymerizing substance we use, which is still in a trial stage, is a fluid silicone oil which is mixed, just prior to use, with a catalyst and a small amount of opacifying tantalum powder; the viscosity of this substance increases after one minute, and it must be rapidly sucked into an insulin syringe (1 cc) with 1/100 graduations, and the proper volume injected immediately.

Since the iodine contrast has a higher density than the polymerizing substance, the inflated balloon will show a lower iodine contrast layer with the slightly opaque silicone oil over it. Once the polymerizing substance has been injected, the tap of the catheter is closed.

In order to release the balloon, the co-axial outer catheter B is brought to the base of the balloon. While doing this, one may feel a certain resistance which could be interpreted as indicating that the outer catheter B has reached the balloon; the operator must then verify if this is so, by measuring the free length of the inner catheter A, which must reach 20 cm, as explained earlier; if not, further advancement of the outer catheter B is required.

At this time, traction is exerted on the inner catheter A (while the outer catheter B is firmly kept in place) and the operator feels clearly the release of the balloon; this step is radioscopically controlled. We must see that the balloon does not move at the time of release.

Both catheters A and B are then withdrawn from the introducer C, and a new arteriographic control (AP and lateral) is carried out.

Three conditions must then be met:

the balloon must be visible in the cavernous sinus, outside the carotid artery;

no leakage of iodine contrast used for arteriogram must occur in the cavernous sinus;

carotid blood flow must be normal.

This technique appears to be the best available although only in our last patients has the silicone oil been used.

Our first patients were treated with balloons inflated with iodine contrast only, a more simple technique; but our experience is that a gradual volume reduction of the balloon occurred during the weeks following the treatment. This of course, cannot occur when using a polymerizing substance. We have successfully treated three aneurysms of the carotid siphon, nine carotid-cavernous sinus fistulas, and two vertebral fistulas (Table 1). All these patients are safe. Two other patients had complications. One had an aneurysm of C 1; he was comatose, grade 4 with a flat E.E.G.; the aneurysm ruptured, while trying to enter the neck with the balloon. The second patient had an aneurysm of the bifurcation of the Sylvian artery. He developed a hemiplegia after the procedure. One branch of the Sylvian artery was occluded, the patient was operated but died some days later. The aim of this paper is to explain this new technique in details and not to present either an exhaustive study of our cases or of the indications of the technique.

Three different examples of the use of this technique are given:

the first one concerns a vertebro-vertebral fistula (Figs. 11 and 12); an iodine inflated balloon has been released in the fistula which is occluded, while the vertebral artery blood flow is maintained (Fig. 13);

the second is of an intra-cavernous aneurysm of the internal carotid artery; an iodine inflated balloon fills the aneurysm (Figs. 14 and 15);

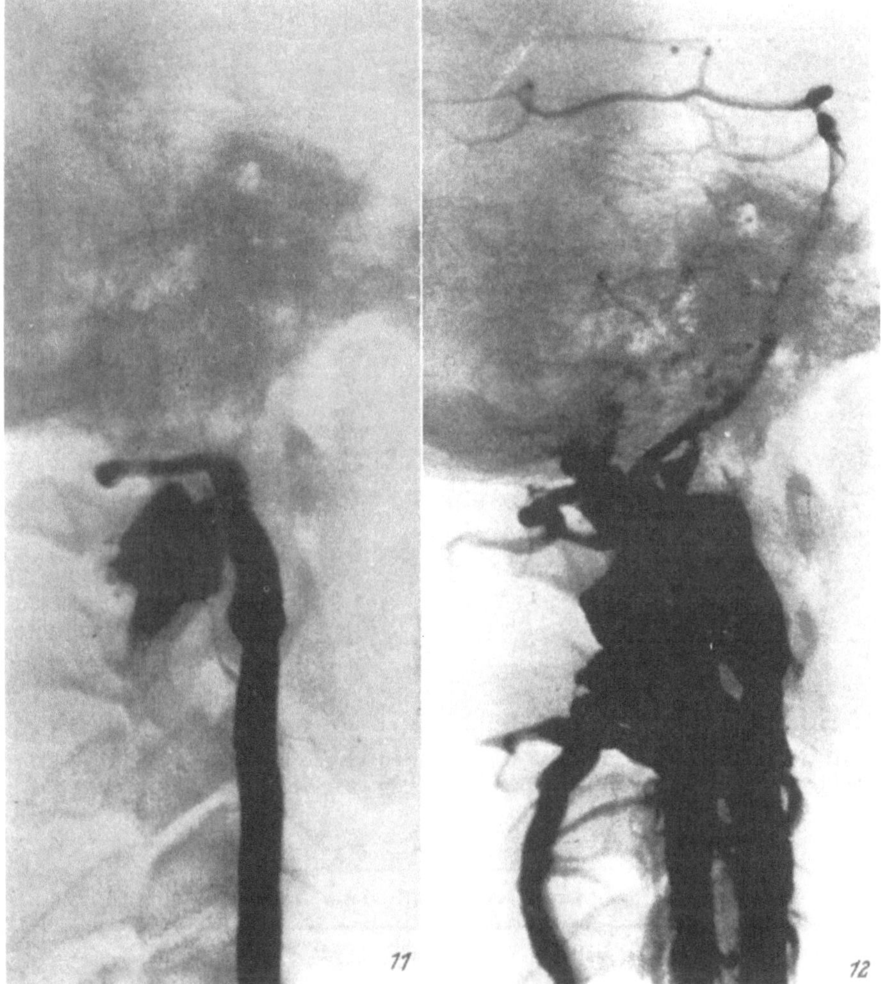

Figs. 11 and 12. Congenital vertebro-vertebral fistula at C 1–C 2

the third example shows a post-traumatic carotid-cavernous fistula (Fig. 16); the balloon has been released in the cavernous sinus; the fistula has disappeared, and carotid flow is normal (Fig. 17).

Conclusion

The technique of an inflatable and releasable balloon finds its best indications in the treatment of post-traumatic carotid-cavernous fistulas. Spontaneous

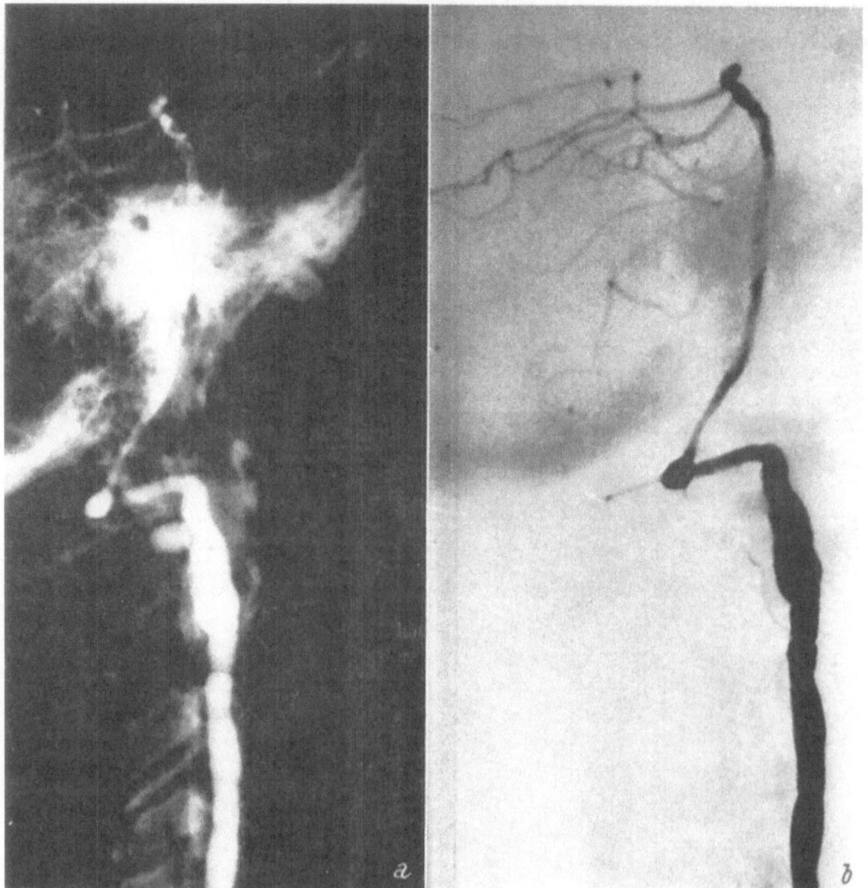

Figs. 13 a and b. The balloon has been released in the fistula and is still opacified eight days later. The fistula is occluded. The vertebral blood flow is preserved

Table 1

Carotid cavernous fistulas	Sem.	Lac.	Gui.	Dra.	Fra.	Bir.	Lac.	Tri.	Fus.
Balloon inflated with contrast and released	+	+	—	—	+	—	+	+	+
Balloon inflated with silicone and released	—	—	+	+	—	+	—	—	—
Carotid blood flow preserved	+	—	+	—	—	+	—	—	+

Vertebro-vertebral fistulas	Lap.	Bab.	Aneurysm of the cavernous portion of the carotid siphon	Sce.	Gui.	Oul.
Balloon inflated with contrast	+	+	Balloon inflated with contrast	+	—	+
Balloon inflated with silicone	—	—	Balloon inflated with silicone	—	+	—
Vertebral flow preserved	+	—	Carotid blood flow preserved	+	+	+

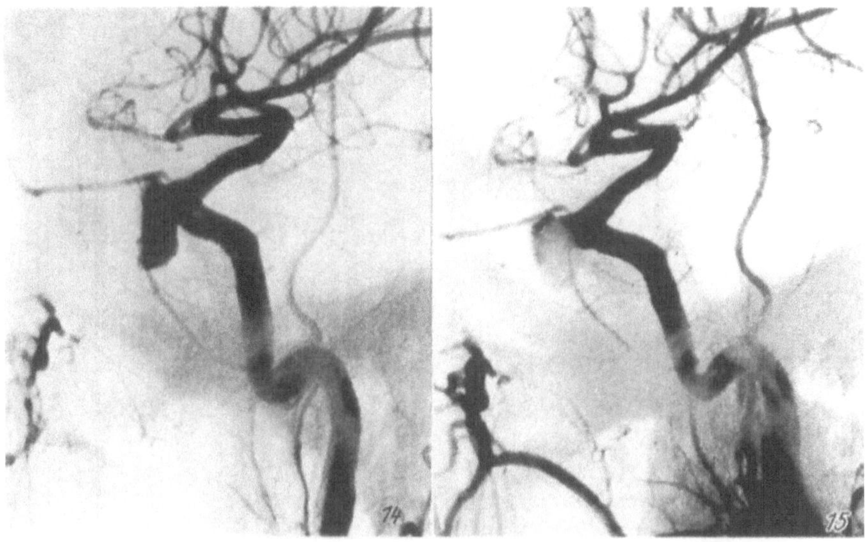

Fig. 14. Aneurysm of the carotid siphon in the cavernous sinus
Fig. 15. One balloon has been released in the aneurysmal pouch which is occluded

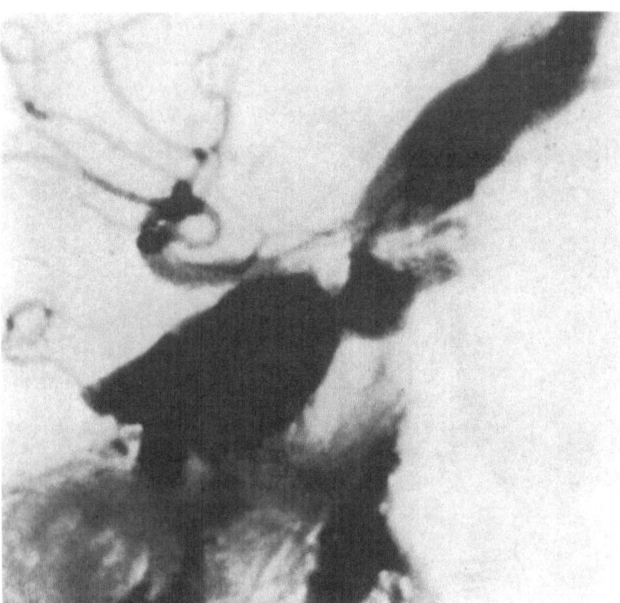

Fig. 16. Post-traumatic carotid-cavernous sinus fistula

carotid-cavernous fistulas are another disease in which many arterial pedicles flow into the cavernous sinus.

As experience has shown to the authors that iodine filled balloons do not keep a constant volume, the use of a polymerizing substance whose volume is permanent, is more satisfactory.

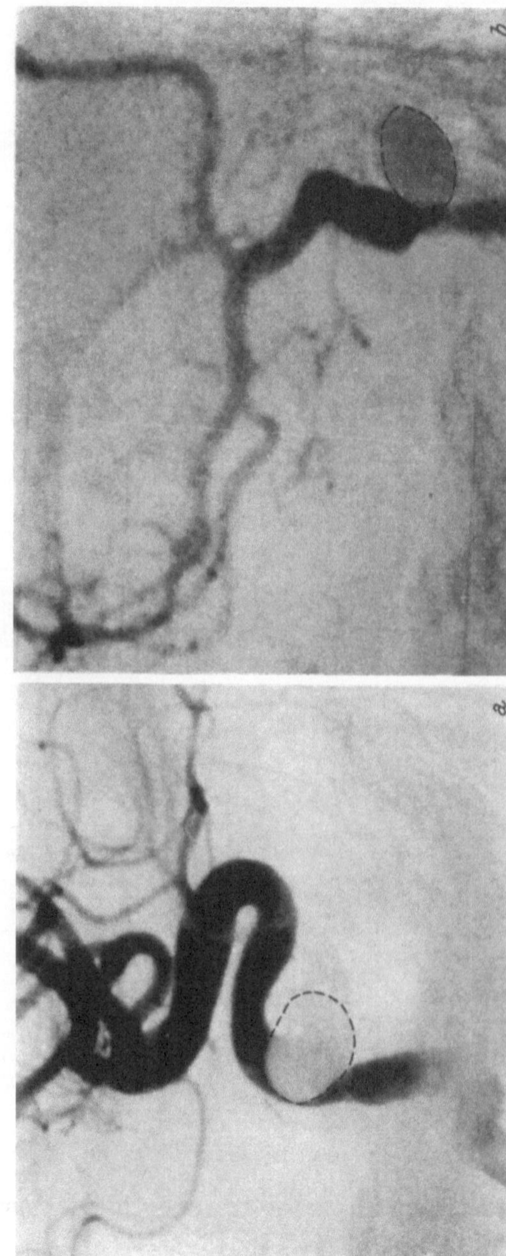

Fig. 17. a) One balloon has been released in the cavernous sinus. The fistula is occluded. The carotid blood flow is preserved; b) on the frontal view the balloon is well seen inside the internal carotid, in the cavernous sinus

A further improvement would consist in dispensing with the co-axial catheter to release the balloon: this could be achieved by using a balloon adapted to the catheter without any ligature, which would be released by a sudden slight traction. We hope to solve this problem soon.

Summary

The technique of an inflatable releasable balloon allows treatment of some intra-cerebral vascular lesions, particularily in the cases of post-traumatic carotid-cavernous fistulas.

This technique involves a small finger-shaped latex sleeve, which is attached to the end of a catheter by an elastic thread, which shuts the balloon when it is released. Release of the balloon is obtained by the use of a co-axial catheter.

The first patients have been treated by iodine contrast inflated balloons; but, as gradual resorption of iodine solution within the following weeks occurs, the use of a polymerizing substance which keeps a permanent volume is preferred.

References

1. Serbinenko, F. A., 1974: Balloon catheterization and occlusion of major cerebral vessels. J. Neurosurg. *41*, 125—145.
2. Debrun, G., Lacour, P., Caron, J. P., Hurth, M., Comoy, J., Keravel, Y., 1975: Experimental approach of carotid-cavernous fistula with an inflatable and isolated balloon, Application in man. Neuroradiol. *9*, 9—12.
3. Debrun, G., Lacour, P., Caron, J. P., Hurth, M., Comoy, J., Keravel, Y., 1975: Inflatable and released balloon technique. Experimentation in dog. Application in man. Neuroradiol. *9*, 267—271.
4. Debrun, G., Lacour, P., Caron, J. P., Hurth, M., Comoy, J., Keravel, Y., Loisance, D., 1975: Traitement de fistules artério-veineuses et d'anévrysmes par ballon gonflable et largable. Bases expérimentales. Application à l'homme. La nouvelle Presse Médicale *4*, 2315—2318.
5. Debrun, G., Lacour, P., Caron, J. P., Hurth, M., Comoy, J., Keravel, Y., Laborit, G., 1975: Technique endovasculaire de ballonnet gonflable et largable. Les Annales de Radiologie *3*, 313—315.
6. Debrun, G., Lacour, P., 1975: Variations sur un thème connu "La Technique de Seldinger". Annales de Radiologie *18*, 761—762.

Author Index

Subject Index

Satz: Adolf Holzhausens Nfg., 1070 Wien
Offsetdruck: Bors & Müller, 1010 Wien

Advances and Technical Standards in Neurosurgery

Volume 2

With 150 partly coloured figures. XI, 217 pages. 1975.

ISBN 3-211-81293-8 (Wien)
ISBN 0-387-81293-8 (New York)

Contents

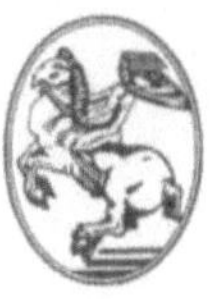

SPRINGER-VERLAG WIEN NEW YORK

Advances and Technical Standards in Neurosurgery

Volume 3

With 77 figures. XI, 154 pages. 1976.

ISBN 3-211-81381-0 (Wien)
ISBN 0-387-81381-0 (New York)

Contents

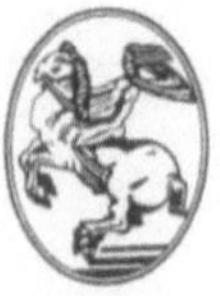

SPRINGER-VERLAG WIEN NEW YORK